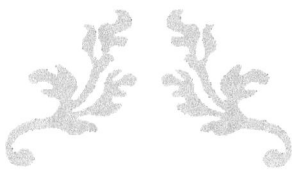

HEALING IN THE BIBLE

Volume 1: Healing in the Old Testament

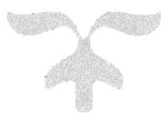

BY J. PITTERSON

Published by Celestial Guide Publications

HEALING IN THE BIBLE
By J. Pitterson

Unless otherwise stated, all scripture quotations are taken from the New King James Version or the King James Version of the Bible.

ISBN 978-1-0698984-1-8 (Paperback)
ISBN 978-1-0698984-2-5 (E-book)
ISBN 978-1-0698984-3-2 (Hardcover)

Copyright © 2025 Celestial Guide Publications
All rights reserved
j.pitterson23@gmail.com

Table of Contents

Introduction 1

PART 1: HEAL IN THE OLD TESTAMENT 9

Chapter 1: Heal in the book of Numbers 10
Chapter 2: Heal in the book of Deuteronomy 16
Chapter 3: Heal in the book of Kings 19
Chapter 4: Heal in the book of Chronicles 22
Chapter 5: Heal in the book of Psalms 25
Chapter 6: Heal in the book of Ecclesiastes 31
Chapter 7: Heal in the book of Isaiah 33
Chapter 8: Heal in the book of Jeremiah 38
Chapter 9: Heal in the book of Lamentations 44
Chapter 10: Heal in the book of Hosea 47
Chapter 11: Heal in the book of Zechariah 53

PART 2: HEALED IN THE OLD TESTAMENT .. 57

Chapter 12: Healed in the book of Genesis 58
Chapter 13: Healed in the book of Exodus 61
Chapter 14: Healed in the book of Leviticus 64
Chapter 15: Healed in the book of Deuteronomy 74
Chapter 16: Healed in the book of Samuel 79
Chapter 17: Healed in the book of Kings 82
Chapter 18: Healed in the book of Chronicles 89
Chapter 19: Healed in the book of Psalms 94
Chapter 20: Healed in the book of Isaiah 98
Chapter 21: Healed in the book of Jeremiah 103
Chapter 22: Healed in the book of Ezekiel 114
Chapter 23: Healed in the book of Hosea 121

PART 3: HEALER IN THE OLD TESTAMENT 127

Chapter 24: Healer in the book of Isaiah 128

PART 4: HEALS IN THE OLD TESTAMENT... 131

Chapter 25: Heals in the book of Exodus................132
Chapter 26: Heals in the book of Psalms 136
Chapter 27: Heals in the book of Isaiah 141

PART 5: HEALING IN THE OLD TESTAMENT 145

Chapter 28: Healing in the book of Jeremiah..........146
Chapter 29: Healing in the book of Nahum 152
Chapter 30: Healing in the book of Malachi............156

PART 6: HEALTH IN THE OLD TESTAMENT 161

Chapter 31: Health in the book of Genesis...............162
Chapter 32: Health in the book of Samuel...............166
Chapter 33: Health in the book of Psalms 170
Chapter 34: Health in the book of Proverbs 178
Chapter 35: Health in the book of Isaiah 191
Chapter 36: Health in the book of Jeremiah............196

Conclusion 211

Special thanks to Prophet Uebert Angel for his mentorship.

Introduction

Healing is one of the most powerful and personal experiences in human life. Whether it's the healing of a body, a broken heart, or a wounded spirit, we all long to be made whole. The Bible speaks often about healing, and while many people focus on the miracles of Jesus in the New Testament, the Old Testament also has much to say about God's healing work. This book explores how healing appears throughout the Old Testament—how it reflects God's character, how it connects to His covenant with His people, and how it points forward to the hope of full restoration.

In the pages of the Old Testament, we find stories of sickness and recovery, of judgment and mercy, of brokenness and renewal. We see God as a healer—not just of physical illness, but of nations, relationships, and hearts. Healing in the Old Testament is not just about medicine or miracles. It's about God's desire to restore what has been damaged by sin, suffering, and separation.

God the Healer: Jehovah Rapha

One of the first names given to God in the Bible is Jehovah Rapha, which means "the Lord who heals." This name appears in Exodus 15:26, where God tells the Israelites, "I am the Lord who heals you." This moment comes after God delivers His people from slavery in Egypt and brings them through the Red Sea. It's a turning point—not just in their journey, but in their understanding of who God is. He is not only a rescuer and provider; He is also a healer.

This name sets the tone for how healing is understood throughout the Old Testament. Healing is not just a physical act—it's a reflection of God's nature. He is compassionate, attentive, and powerful. He sees suffering and responds with mercy. He restores what is broken and brings life where there was death.

Healing and Covenant

Healing in the Old Testament is closely tied to God's covenant with His people. A covenant is a sacred promise, a relationship built on trust and obedience. When Israel follows God's ways, they experience blessing, including health and protection. When they turn away, they often face consequences—sickness, war, and exile.

But even in times of judgment, God's heart remains tender. He sends prophets to call the people back. He offers healing—not just of bodies, but of the land, the community, and the soul. In 2 Chronicles 7:14, God says, "If my people...will humble themselves and pray...I will hear from heaven...and heal their land." This healing is part of the covenant promise. It shows that restoration is always possible when people return to God.

Healing Through Prayer and Intercession

Many healing stories in the Old Testament involve prayer. People cry out to God in times of trouble, and He responds. Abraham prays for Abimelech's household, and God heals them (Genesis 20). Moses pleads for his sister Miriam when she is struck with leprosy, and God shows mercy (Numbers 12). Hannah prays for a child, and her barrenness is healed (1 Samuel 1).

These stories show that healing is not automatic—it often comes through relationship, through faith, and through asking. God listens to the prayers of His people. He responds to their cries. Healing is not just a transaction; it's a conversation between God and those who trust Him.

Healing Through Prophets

In the Old Testament, prophets play a key role in healing. Elijah and Elisha, for example, perform miracles that restore life and health. Elisha heals Naaman, a Syrian commander, of leprosy (2 Kings 5). This story is especially powerful because it shows that healing is not limited to Israelites. God's mercy reaches beyond borders and traditions.

Prophets also speak words of healing. Isaiah, Jeremiah, and Ezekiel all describe God's desire to heal His people—not just physically, but spiritually. Isaiah 53 speaks of the suffering servant who "was pierced for our transgressions...by his wounds we are healed." This passage points forward to Jesus, but it also reflects the deep truth that healing comes through sacrifice and love.

Healing and Holiness

In the Old Testament, health and holiness are often connected. The laws given to Israel include many instructions about cleanliness, disease, and purity. These rules may seem strange to modern readers, but they were meant to protect the community and teach spiritual lessons. Sickness was sometimes seen as a sign of sin or separation from God. Healing, then, was not just about feeling better—it was about being restored to fellowship with God and others.

Leviticus, for example, describes how priests would examine people with skin diseases and declare them clean or unclean. When someone was healed, they would offer sacrifices and be welcomed back into the community. This process shows that healing was both physical and social. It was about being made whole in every way.

Healing and Judgment

Not all sickness in the Old Testament is random. Sometimes, it comes as a result of disobedience. When Israel turns away from God, they face plagues, famine, and disease. These judgments are not meant to destroy—they are meant to call people back to God. In Deuteronomy 28, God lists blessings for obedience and curses for rebellion. Among the curses are illnesses and suffering.

But even in judgment, God offers hope. He says in Hosea 6:1, "Come, let us return to the Lord...He has torn us, but He will heal us." This verse shows that healing is part of God's plan—even when discipline is needed. God does not enjoy punishing His people. He longs to restore them.

Healing and the Future

The Old Testament also looks forward to a time of complete healing. The prophets speak of a day when God will make all things new. Isaiah 35 describes a future where "the eyes of the blind will be opened...the lame will leap like a deer." Ezekiel sees a vision of a river flowing from the temple, bringing life and healing wherever it goes.

These promises point to the coming of the Messiah, who will bring full restoration. They also remind us that healing is not just for the past—it's part of God's future plan. The Old Testament lays the foundation for the hope we find in Jesus, who fulfills these promises and brings healing to the world.

Healing and Community

Healing in the Old Testament is not just personal—it's communal. When one person is healed, the whole community rejoices. When the land is healed, the people thrive. Restoration is meant to be shared. God's healing work brings people together, rebuilds relationships, and strengthens society.

Psalm 147:3 says, "He heals the brokenhearted and binds up their wounds." This verse speaks to emotional and spiritual healing. It shows that God cares about every part of our pain. He doesn't just fix problems—He comforts, restores, and renews.

Healing and Worship

Healing often leads to worship. When people experience God's mercy, they respond with praise. The Psalms are full of songs that celebrate healing. Psalm 103 says, "Bless the Lord...who heals all your diseases." Worship is a natural response to healing. It's a way of saying thank you, of recognizing God's goodness, and of sharing the joy with others.

In the Old Testament, healing is not just a private experience—it's part of the life of faith. It draws people closer to God and invites them to live in gratitude and trust.

A God Who Heals

The Old Testament shows us a God who heals. He heals bodies, hearts, communities, and nations. He responds to prayer, sends prophets, and offers hope. His healing is not limited by time, place, or circumstance. It flows from His love, His covenant, and His desire to restore what is broken.

As we explore healing in the Old Testament, we discover that it is more than a theme—it is a thread that runs through the entire story of Scripture. It reveals God's character, His compassion, and His plan for redemption. It prepares us to understand the healing ministry of Jesus and the ongoing work of the Holy Spirit.

This book will walk through key passages, stories, and teachings about healing in the Old Testament. It will look at how God works in times of sickness and suffering, how He calls people to faith and obedience, and how He brings restoration through mercy and grace. Whether you are seeking healing yourself or simply want to understand God's heart more deeply, this journey through Scripture will offer insight, encouragement, and hope.

Healing is not just something God does—it's part of who He is. And the Old Testament invites us to know Him as the One who heals.

Your comments and suggestions are important to us. Please send them to: j.pitterson23@gmail.com.

PART 1

HEAL IN THE OLD TESTAMENT

Chapter 1
Heal in the book of Numbers

1. Numbers 12:9-15

9 So the anger of the Lord was aroused against them, and He departed.

10 And when the cloud departed from above the tabernacle, suddenly Miriam became leprous, as white as snow. Then Aaron turned toward Miriam, and there she was, a leper.

11 So Aaron said to Moses, "Oh, my lord! Please do not lay this sin on us, in which we have done foolishly and in which we have sinned.

12 Please do not let her be as one dead, whose flesh is half consumed when he comes out of his mother's womb!"

13 So Moses cried out to the Lord, saying, "Please heal her, O God, I pray!"

14 Then the Lord said to Moses, "If her father had but spit in her face, would she not be shamed seven days? Let her be shut out of the camp seven days, and afterward she may be received again."

15 So Miriam was shut out of the camp seven days, and the people did not journey till Miriam was brought in again.

Summary

This passage from Numbers 12 recounts a pivotal moment in Israel's wilderness journey—a confrontation involving Miriam and Aaron, the siblings of Moses, that challenges the spiritual leadership God has established. Their complaint centers on Moses' marriage to a Cushite woman, which they view as a breach of cultural or religious norms. However, the deeper issue is not the marriage itself, but jealousy over Moses' unique relationship with God.

Miriam and Aaron question Moses' authority, implying that they too receive divine revelation and should share leadership. Their challenge is not just personal—it threatens the spiritual order God has put in place. In response, the Lord visibly descends in a pillar of cloud and summons all three to the tent of meeting, the sacred space where God speaks with His people.

There, God speaks with unmistakable clarity. He affirms Moses' singular role, declaring that while other prophets receive dreams and visions, Moses speaks with God "face to face," with clarity and intimacy. This is not only a defense of Moses—it is a rebuke to Miriam and Aaron for undermining God's chosen servant. God's anger flares, and He departs from the tent. As the cloud lifts, Miriam is suddenly afflicted with leprosy.

The text suggests that Miriam's affliction is not a direct strike from God, but a consequence of His anger—a withdrawal of divine protection that leaves her exposed to judgment. In biblical times, leprosy was more than a disease; it symbolized spiritual impurity and social exclusion. Miriam's condition immediately marks her as unclean, and she accepts her punishment without protest, acknowledging her role in the rebellion.

Aaron, witnessing the severity of her condition, turns to Moses in desperation. He confesses their sin and pleads for mercy on Miriam's behalf. Moved by compassion, Moses offers one of the most heartfelt prayers in Scripture: "Heal her, O God, I pray." This is the first recorded instance in the Bible where the word "heal" is used in a direct plea to God.

The Hebrew word translated as "heal" here is *raphah*, a term rich in meaning. While often associated with physical healing, *raphah* encompasses a broader spectrum of restoration:

- **Physical relaxation**: To become limp or fall, suggesting a release from tension or affliction.
- **Emotional surrender**: To cease striving, to let go of control, and to yield to divine intervention.

- **Stillness**: To be silent, to stop resisting, and to enter a state of peace.
- **Withdrawal**: To disengage from a struggle or remove oneself from harm.

In the context of Moses' prayer, *raphah* carries the sense of "withdrawal." Moses is not simply asking for a cure—he is pleading with God to withdraw His judgment from Miriam. He recognizes that her leprosy is not a random illness, but a direct result of divine displeasure. His prayer is a request for God to relent, to restore Miriam, and to reintegrate her into the community.

God responds with both justice and mercy. He instructs that Miriam be isolated outside the camp for seven days—a period of purification and reflection. This mirrors the cultural practice of distancing someone who has been dishonored, as if her father had spat in her face—a metaphor used in the text to express the depth of her shame. Yet this isolation is not permanent. It is a path to healing, a space for restoration. After seven days, Miriam is healed and welcomed back into the community.

This passage offers several profound theological insights:

- **Divine Order and Authority.** God's defense of Moses highlights the importance of respecting divinely appointed leadership. Challenges rooted in pride or jealousy disrupt the spiritual harmony of the community. God's response is swift and decisive, reaffirming the sacred nature of Moses' role and the seriousness of undermining it.

- **The Nature of Divine Healing.** The introduction of raphah marks a significant moment in biblical theology. Healing is not just physical—it is the withdrawal of judgment, the restoration of wholeness, and the return to divine favor. Moses' prayer reveals the power of intercession and the compassion that should accompany spiritual leadership.

- **The Consequences of Provoking Divine Anger.** Miriam's leprosy serves as a cautionary example. While God is merciful, His anger has real consequences. The passage reminds us that rebellion against divine order can result in affliction—not necessarily as punishment, but as the natural outcome of stepping outside God's protective boundaries.

- **Restoration Through Repentance and Intercession.** Miriam's acceptance of her punishment, Aaron's plea for mercy, and Moses' intercessory prayer form a model of communal repentance. Healing and restoration are possible when there is humility, acknowledgment of wrongdoing, and a sincere appeal to God's mercy.

In conclusion, this passage is a powerful narrative of leadership, judgment, and grace. It reveals the seriousness of challenging God's appointed servants, the depth of divine compassion, and the transformative power of prayer. The use of *raphah* introduces a theology of healing that encompasses physical, emotional, and spiritual dimensions—reminding us that restoration begins when we surrender to God and seek His mercy.

Chapter 2
Heal in the book of Deuteronomy

1. Deuteronomy 32:36-39

36 "For the Lord will judge His people And have compassion on His servants, When He sees that their power is gone, And there is no one remaining, bond or free.

37 He will say: 'Where are their gods, The rock in which they sought refuge?

38 Who ate the fat of their sacrifices, And drank the wine of their drink offering? Let them rise and help you, And be your refuge.

39 'Now see that I, even I, am He, And there is no God besides Me; I kill and I make alive; I wound and I heal; Nor is there any who can deliver from My hand.

Summary

This passage from Deuteronomy 32 presents a moment of divine confrontation and mercy. Speaking on behalf of God, Moses announces judgment against Israel for their idolatry—offering sacrifices to foreign gods and seeking refuge in powerless deities. These idols, once trusted in times of prosperity, are exposed as empty and ineffective. God declares that when His people are broken and abandoned, He will ask, "Where are your gods now—the ones who consumed your offerings?"

This rhetorical question reveals the futility of idolatry. The gods Israel once honored will be silent in their time of need. In contrast, God asserts His unmatched authority:

"See now that I, even I, am He, and there is no god besides Me; I put to death and I bring to life, I wound and I heal, and no one can deliver out of My hand."

This declaration affirms several foundational truths. First, God alone is sovereign—no other power shares His authority. Second, He holds complete control over life and death, judgment and restoration. His actions are final, and His will cannot be challenged. Yet even in judgment, God's mercy remains. When He sees His people weary and broken, He responds with compassion. His mercy is not earned—it flows from His character.

The word "heal" in this passage is especially meaningful. It comes from the Hebrew root *rapha*, which can appear in two forms:

- *raphah* (הִפָּרֵ): meaning to relax, let go, or become weak—often used to describe surrender or stillness.

- *rapha* (אָפָךְ): meaning to heal, restore, or repair—used to describe active and complete restoration.

In this context, the meaning clearly supports *rapha*, emphasizing God's role as the Healer. He does not merely allow suffering to fade—He actively restores what is broken. His healing is full, reaching into every part of human need: physical, emotional, spiritual, and communal.

This passage highlights several key themes:

- **God's Sovereignty**: He alone governs life, death, and healing.
- **God's Compassion**: Even after rebellion, He remains ready to restore.
- **The Power of Divine Healing**: Restoration is real, deep, and transformative.
- **The Call to Trust**: Idols fail, but God remains faithful and powerful.

Ultimately, this text calls believers to trust in God alone—not only in times of blessing, but especially in moments of crisis and repentance. His healing is complete, and His grace is enduring. God wounds, but He also heals—and when He heals, He restores with fullness and mercy.

Chapter 3
Heal in the book of Kings

1. 2 Kings 20:5-8

5 "Return and tell Hezekiah the leader of My people, 'Thus says the Lord, the God of David your father: "I have heard your prayer, I have seen your tears; surely I will heal you. On the third day you shall go up to the house of the Lord.

6 And I will add to your days fifteen years. I will deliver you and this city from the hand of the king of Assyria; and I will defend this city for My own sake, and for the sake of My servant David." ' "

7 Then Isaiah said, "Take a lump of figs." So they took and laid it on the boil, and he recovered.

8 And Hezekiah said to Isaiah, "What is the sign that the Lord will heal me, and that I shall go up to the house of the Lord the third day?"

Summary

This passage from the book of Isaiah recounts a deeply moving moment in the life of King Hezekiah. Critically ill and facing death, Hezekiah receives a solemn message from the prophet Isaiah: he must prepare his household, for his life is nearing its end. Confronted with this grave news, Hezekiah turns to God in earnest prayer, appealing to his years of faithful service, wholehearted devotion, and righteous living. His plea is sincere, personal, and filled with humility.

Before Isaiah has even left the palace, God responds. He instructs the prophet to return with a new message: Hezekiah will be healed, and his life extended by fifteen years. In addition, God promises to deliver both Hezekiah and Jerusalem from the threat of the Assyrian king, reaffirming His covenant with David and the holiness of His name.

Isaiah then orders a poultice of figs to be applied to Hezekiah's ulcer, leading to his physical recovery. As confirmation of this divine promise, God performs a miraculous sign—the shadow on the sundial moves backward ten degrees, symbolizing not only the reversal of time but the restoration of life.

This passage powerfully demonstrates God's responsiveness to heartfelt prayer, His compassion for those who seek Him, and His sovereign control over life, healing, and protection. The Hebrew word used for "heal" in this context is *rapha*, which means to cure, restore, or make whole. It signifies more than physical recovery—it points to complete healing that touches body, soul, and spirit. *Rapha* reflects God's nature as the ultimate healer, one who not only removes affliction but restores fullness and peace.

Hezekiah's story reminds us that divine mercy can reach into the darkest moments. His healing was not earned through ritual or status, but through sincere prayer rooted in trust and humility. It shows that God listens, responds, and acts with grace when His people call on Him.

Ultimately, this passage affirms that healing in the biblical sense is holistic. It is not limited to physical wellness but includes emotional renewal, spiritual restoration, and divine protection. Through *rapha*, we see that God's healing is intentional, complete, and deeply personal—an expression of His love and power to restore what is broken.

Chapter 4
Heal in the book of Chronicles

1. 2 Chronicles 7:12-14

12 Then the Lord appeared to Solomon by night, and said to him: "I have heard your prayer, and have chosen this place for Myself as a house of sacrifice.

13 When I shut up heaven and there is no rain, or command the locusts to devour the land, or send pestilence among My people,

14 if My people who are called by My name will humble themselves, and pray and seek My face, and turn from their wicked ways, then I will hear from heaven, and will forgive their sin and heal their land.

Summary

This passage, drawn from the aftermath of Solomon's prayer at the temple dedication, marks a profound moment of divine affirmation. God appears to Solomon in a dream, confirming that He has heard the prayer and has chosen the temple as His sacred dwelling—a place set apart for worship, sacrifice, and communion with His people.

More than a spiritual center, God designates the temple as a place of restoration. He declares that when drought, pestilence, or other hardships come as discipline, the people may return to this holy place to seek Him. If they humble themselves, pray, pursue His presence, and turn from their sinful ways, He will respond with mercy. God promises to forgive their sins and heal their land, restoring both spiritual vitality and physical well-being.

This passage offers a striking theological insight: healing is not limited to individuals. The land itself—impacted by human disobedience—can suffer and be restored. Divine healing, in this context, reaches beyond personal affliction to touch entire communities and environments. The restoration of the land is directly tied to repentance and renewed relationship with God.

The Hebrew word translated as "heal" is *rapha*, which means to cure, repair, or restore. In this passage, *rapha* conveys more than physical recovery—it signifies divine intervention that mends what is broken, whether in the human heart or the land itself. It reflects God's desire not only to forgive but to renew, bringing wholeness where there was once damage.

Ultimately, this passage underscores God's responsiveness to sincere prayer, His compassion toward a repentant people, and His power to restore what has been harmed. The temple becomes a symbol of hope—a place where healing begins through humility, prayer, and transformation. It reminds us that restoration is possible when we turn back to God, and that His healing is complete, reaching into every dimension of life.

Chapter 5
Heal in the book of Psalms

1. Psalm 6:1-2

1 O Lord, do not rebuke me in Your anger, Nor chasten me in Your hot displeasure.

2 Have mercy on me, O Lord, for I am weak; O Lord, heal me, for my bones are troubled.

Summary

This passage reveals a deeply intimate and vulnerable moment in King David's life, as he cries out to God during a time of intense suffering. Whether his pain is physical, emotional, or spiritual, David pleads with the Lord not to rebuke him in anger or discipline him in wrath. His prayer is marked by humility and honesty, acknowledging his weakness and appealing to God's compassion.

David's request for healing goes beyond seeking relief from pain—it is a heartfelt plea for restoration and reconciliation. He understands that only God can repair what is broken within him. His words reflect a deep dependence on divine mercy and a trust that God's goodness will prevail, even in the midst of judgment. David's posture of surrender shows spiritual maturity; he does not defend himself or demand deliverance, but submits to God's will while asking for grace.

The Hebrew word translated as "heal" in this passage is *rapha*, a verb rich in meaning. It signifies more than curing physical illness—it encompasses the act of repairing, restoring, and making whole. In this context, *rapha* speaks to a holistic healing that reaches every part of David's being. He longs for restoration not only of his body, but of his soul and his relationship with God.

This moment in Scripture highlights key aspects of David's character: his awareness of human frailty, his humility before God, and his unwavering trust in divine mercy. It offers a timeless reminder that true healing begins with honest prayer, repentance, and a heart fully surrendered to the One who heals.

Ultimately, this passage affirms that God's healing is not limited to physical recovery. Through *rapha*, we see that divine restoration touches the whole person—body, mind, and spirit. David's cry invites all believers to approach God with humility, trusting that His mercy can restore what is broken and renew what has been lost.

2. Psalm 41:1-4

1 Blessed is he who considers the poor; The Lord will deliver him in time of trouble.

2 The Lord will preserve him and keep him alive, And he will be blessed on the earth; You will not deliver him to the will of his enemies.

3 The Lord will strengthen him on his bed of illness; You will sustain him on his sickbed.

4 I said, "Lord, be merciful to me; Heal my soul, for I have sinned against You."

Summary

This passage from Psalm 41 reflects King David's affirmation of God's special care for those who show kindness to the poor and vulnerable. He declares that such individuals are blessed by God, who promises to protect them in times of trouble, preserve their lives, and guard them from the harm intended by their enemies. In times of sickness, God will sustain them, offering strength, comfort, and restoration.

David then moves from public declaration to personal prayer. In a moment of self-reflection, he turns to God with humility, acknowledging his own sin and pleading for mercy. His request—"heal my soul"—reveals a deep awareness of his spiritual need and a profound trust in God's power to restore. This plea is not simply for physical healing, but for inner renewal, reconciliation, and wholeness.

The Hebrew word translated as "heal" in this passage is *rapha*, a rich and layered term that means to heal, repair, or make whole. In this context, *rapha* expresses David's longing for complete restoration—not only of his body, but of his soul and relationship with God. It reflects the biblical view that true healing touches every part of life: physical, emotional, and spiritual.

This passage also highlights the close connection between compassion and divine favor. David's words suggest that those who care for others in their weakness will themselves be cared for by God in their time of need. His prayer reveals his dependence on divine mercy and his confidence in the healing that flows from a relationship rooted in grace.

Ultimately, this psalm affirms that God's healing is not limited to the body. Through *rapha*, we see that God restores the whole person—healing not only visible wounds but also the hidden pain of the heart. David's prayer invites all who are weary or broken to seek God with sincerity and faith, trusting that He is both willing and able to restore what has been lost.

3. Psalm 60:1-2

1 O God, You have cast us off; You have broken us down; You have been displeased; Oh, restore us again!

2 You have made the earth tremble; You have broken it; Heal its breaches, for it is shaking.

Summary

This passage from Psalm 60 captures King David's heartfelt plea to God during a time of national crisis, likely amid military conflict involving Israel, Mesopotamia, and Syria. Confronted by defeat and instability, David turns to God in lament, acknowledging the deep wounds suffered by the nation. He describes Israel as shaken, broken, and disoriented under divine judgment, sensing God's apparent withdrawal and the crumbling of its foundations.

Yet David's prayer is not one of despair—it is filled with hope rooted in faith. He appeals to God's mercy and sovereignty, asking for restoration and guidance. His words reflect a deep understanding that healing and renewal can only come from God, even when hardship is the result of divine discipline. David does not seek relief through military strength or political strategy; he seeks healing through divine intervention.

The Hebrew word translated as "heal" in this passage is *rapha*, a term rich in meaning. It signifies more than physical recovery—it includes repairing, restoring, and making whole. In this context, *rapha* conveys the idea of national restoration. David is asking God to mend not just physical damage, but the spiritual and communal integrity of Israel. The use of *rapha* emphasizes that true healing comes from God alone, who can restore what has been broken—whether in the heart of a person or the life of a nation.

This passage reveals David's unwavering trust in God's authority, even in moments of judgment. It affirms that divine healing is not limited to curing illness but extends to rebuilding communities, renewing spiritual identity, and restoring peace.

HEALING IN THE BIBLE

David's prayer models humility, dependence, and confidence in God's redemptive power.

Ultimately, Psalm 60 reminds us that healing begins with honest prayer and a return to God. Through *rapha*, we see that restoration is possible—not just for individuals, but for entire nations—when people turn back to the One who heals with grace, completeness, and compassion.

Chapter 6
Heal in the book of Ecclesiastes

1. Ecclesiastes 3:1-3

1 To everything there is a season, A time for every purpose under heaven:

2 A time to be born, And a time to die; A time to plant, And a time to pluck what is planted;

3 A time to kill, And a time to heal; A time to break down, And a time to build up;

Summary

This passage from Ecclesiastes 3 offers Solomon's thoughtful reflection on the seasons of life and God's divine control over time. He begins with the powerful statement that "there is a time for everything," emphasizing that every part of human experience unfolds according to a divine rhythm. Life moves in cycles—birth and death, joy and sorrow, building and breaking—all under God's sovereign direction.

Solomon illustrates this truth through a series of contrasts that reflect the natural flow of life: "a time to be born and a time to die" captures the full span of human existence; "a time to plant and a time to uproot" speaks to growth and change; "a time to kill and a time to heal" highlights the tension between destruction and restoration; and "a time to tear down and a time to build" points to the ongoing process of renewal. These examples remind us that change is inevitable and that wisdom lies in recognizing and responding to each season with humility.

The passage invites readers to acknowledge that every moment—whether joyful or painful—has meaning within God's greater plan. Life is not random or chaotic; it is shaped by a Creator who appoints times for loss, growth, healing, and rebuilding. Trusting in this divine timing brings peace, even when circumstances are difficult or unclear.

The word "heal" in this passage is translated from the Hebrew *rapha*, which means to heal, restore, or make whole. In this context, *rapha* conveys the idea of deep restoration—repairing what has been broken and renewing what has been harmed. Solomon's use of this word affirms that healing is not only possible, but purposeful. It reflects God's desire to bring wholeness, even after seasons of conflict or loss.

Ultimately, this passage encourages us to trust in God's timing and to find peace in the rhythm of life He has ordained. Through *rapha*, we are reminded that healing is part of the divine cycle—a promise that restoration will come, and that every season, no matter how difficult, is held within the hands of a faithful and sovereign God.

Chapter 7
Heal in the book of Isaiah

1. Isaiah 19:18-22

18 In that day five cities in the land of Egypt will speak the language of Canaan and swear by the Lord of hosts; one will be called the City of Destruction.

19 In that day there will be an altar to the Lord in the midst of the land of Egypt, and a pillar to the Lord at its border.

20 And it will be for a sign and for a witness to the Lord of hosts in the land of Egypt; for they will cry to the Lord because of the oppressors, and He will send them a Savior and a Mighty One, and He will deliver them.

21 Then the Lord will be known to Egypt, and the Egyptians will know the Lord in that day, and will make sacrifice and offering; yes, they will make a vow to the Lord and perform it.

22 And the Lord will strike Egypt, He will strike and heal it; they will return to the Lord, and He will be entreated by them and heal them.

Summary

This passage from the prophetic writings of Isaiah presents a powerful vision of transformation and redemption for Egypt. Rather than remaining a distant or adversarial nation in biblical history, Egypt is portrayed as a future participant in worship and covenant with the God of Israel. Isaiah foresees a time when Egypt, once marked by idolatry and oppression, will experience a spiritual awakening and turn fully to the Lord.

The prophecy begins with a striking image: five cities in Egypt will speak the language of Canaan and pledge allegiance to the God of Israel. This shift in language and loyalty symbolizes a deep cultural and spiritual change. One of these cities will be called the "City of Destruction," likely reflecting its journey from ruin to renewal—a place once broken, now restored.

During this time, an altar to the Lord will be built in the heart of Egypt. More than a symbol, it will serve as a center of worship, sacrifice, and covenantal devotion. The Egyptians, weighed down by oppression, will cry out to God, and He will respond by sending a savior to deliver them. This divine intervention marks a turning point in Egypt's spiritual story.

As the Lord becomes known among the Egyptians, they will begin to offer sacrifices, make vows, and fulfill them—demonstrating sincere commitment and reverence. Isaiah then reveals a profound truth:

though the Lord will strike Egypt, He will also heal it. The affliction is a form of discipline, but it leads to restoration. The people will return to God in repentance, and He will respond with healing.

The Hebrew word used for "heal" in this passage is *rapha*, meaning to heal, repair, or make whole. In this context, *rapha* expresses the full scope of divine restoration—physical, spiritual, and communal. It reflects God's desire not only to correct but to renew, drawing Egypt into the community of worshipers and restoring its place in His redemptive plan.

Ultimately, this prophecy reveals a future in which Egypt experiences both judgment and grace. It becomes a living testimony to God's mercy and power to restore. No nation is beyond His reach, and healing is always possible when hearts turn toward Him. Through *rapha*, Isaiah affirms that God's restoration is complete, compassionate, and transformative.

2. Isaiah 57:16-21

16 For I will not contend forever, Nor will I always be angry; For the spirit would fail before Me, And the souls which I have made.

17 For the iniquity of his covetousness I was angry and struck him; I hid and was angry, And he went on backsliding in the way of his heart.

18 I have seen his ways, and will heal him; I will also lead him, And restore comforts to him And to his mourners.

19 "I create the fruit of the lips: Peace, peace to him who is far off and to him who is near," Says the Lord, "And I will heal him."

20 But the wicked are like the troubled sea, When it cannot rest, Whose waters cast up mire and dirt.

21 "There is no peace," Says my God, "for the wicked."

Summary

This passage from the prophetic writings of Isaiah presents a powerful message from God to the people of Israel, who had turned away from Him through idolatry and spiritual rebellion. Speaking through the prophet, God confronts the nation with the reality of their sin, reminding them that their actions carry consequences. His justice demands accountability, and His anger—provoked by persistent greed and defiance—cannot be ignored. Yet, even in judgment, God's message is not one of condemnation alone, but of hope and restoration.

God declares that His anger will not last forever. Though His people have resisted correction and continued in their wrongdoing, He reveals that His mercy ultimately surpasses His wrath. In a profound act of compassion, God chooses to respond not with destruction, but with healing. This change is not a sign of inconsistency, but of divine love—a love that seeks to restore rather than punish. He announces His intention to heal His people, to guide them again, and to comfort those who are suffering.

This healing is not limited to physical recovery. It includes spiritual renewal, emotional restoration, and the rebuilding of relationship between God and His people. God extends peace to those who are far away and to those who are near, showing that His grace is inclusive and available to all who turn to Him. The promise to "heal" is rooted in the Hebrew word *rapha*, which means to heal, repair, or make whole. In this context, *rapha* speaks to the complete restoration of Israel—both as individuals and as a community.

However, the passage also presents a clear contrast. For the wicked—described as a restless sea stirring up mud and debris—there will be no peace. This vivid imagery reflects the chaos and instability that come from living apart from God, highlighting the consequences of unrepentant rebellion.

Ultimately, this passage reveals the heart of divine mercy. God is a righteous judge who disciplines, but He is also a compassionate healer who restores. He confronts sin, but He never abandons His people. Through *rapha*, Isaiah affirms that healing is always possible when hearts turn back to God—a healing that brings peace, wholeness, and renewed relationship.

Chapter 8
Heal in the book of Jeremiah

1. Jeremiah 3:20-22

20 Surely, as a wife treacherously departs from her husband, So have you dealt treacherously with Me, O house of Israel," says the Lord.

21 A voice was heard on the desolate heights, Weeping and supplications of the children of Israel. For they have perverted their way; They have forgotten the Lord their God.

22 "Return, you backsliding children, And I will heal your backslidings." "Indeed we do come to You, For You are the Lord our God.

Summary

This passage from the book of Jeremiah addresses the deep spiritual unfaithfulness of Israel and Judah. Through the prophet, God confronts the seriousness of their betrayal, comparing their disloyalty to that of a wife who has broken her marriage vows. This metaphor highlights the personal and relational nature of their sin—a violation of a covenant built on love, trust, and faithfulness.

Despite their rebellion, the people eventually cry out to God from the barren heights—a place that symbolizes their spiritual emptiness and distance from Him. Their lament is genuine. They confess their sins, express sorrow for turning away, and acknowledge the brokenness of their ways. This moment of repentance becomes a turning point, opening the way for divine mercy and restoration.

In response to their sincere contrition, God does not reject them. Instead, He extends an invitation to return and promises healing for their unfaithfulness. This promise is not just symbolic—it reflects God's enduring commitment to His people and His desire to renew the relationship that has been damaged. The people, moved by this offer of grace, respond with a willingness to be reconciled, showing their longing to be restored to fellowship with the Lord.

The Hebrew word translated as "heal" in this passage is *rapha*, a term rich in meaning. It includes the ideas of healing, repairing, and making whole. In this context, *rapha* refers to spiritual restoration—a healing that reaches beyond physical recovery to touch the heart, the soul, and the covenantal bond between God and His people. It speaks to the renewal of trust, the mending of broken relationships, and the reestablishment of divine communion.

Ultimately, this passage reveals the depth of God's compassion. It affirms His readiness to forgive, His unwavering love, and His power to restore those who return to Him with humility and sincerity. Through *rapha*, we see that healing is not just about removing pain—it is about renewing life, rebuilding connection, and restoring wholeness. God's invitation to return is a call to be healed, not only in body, but in spirit and relationship.

2. Jeremiah 17:14-17

14 Heal me, O Lord, and I shall be healed; Save me, and I shall be saved, For You are my praise.

15 Indeed they say to me, "Where is the word of the Lord? Let it come now!"

16 As for me, I have not hurried away from being a shepherd who follows You, Nor have I desired the woeful day; You know what came out of my lips; It was right there before You.

17 Do not be a terror to me; You are my hope in the day of doom.

Summary

This passage, drawn from a deeply personal prayer of the prophet Jeremiah, reveals his earnest appeal to God for healing and salvation. In the midst of suffering and public ridicule, Jeremiah acknowledges that God alone is his source of deliverance and praise. Surrounded by opposition, he faces taunts from enemies who question the presence and power of the God he serves, casting doubt on the legitimacy of his prophetic mission.

Despite these challenges, Jeremiah reaffirms his unwavering commitment to his calling. He reminds God of his faithfulness as a shepherd to the people, consistently proclaiming the divine message without compromise. He emphasizes that he has never sought revenge or rejoiced in the downfall of his adversaries. His appeal is not driven by bitterness, but by a longing for justice and spiritual renewal—for himself and for the people he serves.

Jeremiah's prayer is marked by vulnerability and trust. He pleads not to be abandoned or crushed under the weight of persecution, seeking refuge in God's mercy and protection. His words reflect the inner struggle of a prophet who feels the pain of rejection, yet remains anchored in faith. He does not ask for escape, but for strength to endure and continue his mission with clarity and courage.

The Hebrew word translated as "heal" in this passage is *rapha*, a term that means to heal, repair, or make whole. In this context, *rapha* signifies more than physical recovery—it speaks to the restoration of Jeremiah's spirit, emotional resilience, and sense of purpose. His plea for healing is a request for divine renewal, a restoration that enables him to rise above adversity and remain faithful to his calling.

Ultimately, this passage reveals the depth of Jeremiah's relationship with God—a bond shaped by obedience, tested by hardship, and sustained by hope. It affirms that even in moments of despair, healing is possible through divine grace. The use of *rapha* reminds us that God's restoration reaches beyond the body to the heart and soul, renewing strength and restoring purpose. Jeremiah's prayer stands as a timeless example of faith under pressure, and of the healing that comes when we entrust our brokenness to the One who makes us whole.

3. Jeremiah 30:16-17

16 'Therefore all those who devour you shall be devoured; And all your adversaries, every one of them, shall go into captivity; Those who plunder you shall become plunder, And all who prey upon you I will make a prey.

17 For I will restore health to you And heal you of your wounds,' says the Lord, 'Because they called you an outcast saying: "This is Zion; No one seeks her."'

Summary

This passage from the prophetic writings of Jeremiah speaks to the deep suffering of Israel and Judah, who mourn the severity of their wounds and afflictions. Their cries reflect a nation burdened by pain and loss. In response, God reminds them that their suffering is not random—it is the result of their repeated disobedience and moral failure. Their spiritual rebellion has led to national distress, and the weight of their sins has brought about divine judgment.

Yet even in this moment of rebuke, God reveals His unwavering commitment to both justice and mercy. He declares that those who have oppressed and exploited His people will face consequences. The adversaries of Israel will be taken into captivity, bearing the weight of their own wrongdoing. This reversal of fortunes affirms God's justice and His protection of the covenant people.

More importantly, God offers a promise of restoration. Though Israel has been labeled "outcasts" by others, God does not abandon them. He pledges to restore their health and bind up their wounds—a powerful image of healing and renewal. This assurance goes beyond physical recovery; it speaks to spiritual reconciliation and the rebuilding of national identity.

The Hebrew word translated as "heal" in this passage is *rapha*, a word rich in meaning. It signifies healing, repairing, and making whole. In this context, *rapha* conveys the full scope of divine restoration—touching body, soul, and community. It reflects God's intention to mend what has been broken and to reestablish His people with dignity and strength.

Ultimately, this passage highlights the balance between divine justice and compassion. God confronts sin with truth, but He responds to repentance with healing. His mercy is not weakened by judgment; rather, it is revealed in His willingness to restore those who turn back to Him. Through *rapha*, we see that healing is not just relief from suffering—it is the renewal of relationship, identity, and purpose.

This message offers hope to all who feel wounded or cast aside. It affirms that restoration is possible, even after failure, and that God's healing reaches into every part of life. When His people return with humility, He responds with grace, binding up their wounds and making them whole again.

Chapter 9
Heal in the book of Lamentations

1. Lamentations 2:11-13

11 My eyes fail with tears, My heart is troubled; My bile is poured on the ground Because of the destruction of the daughter of my people, Because the children and the infants Faint in the streets of the city.

12 They say to their mothers, "Where is grain and wine?" As they swoon like the wounded In the streets of the city, As their life is poured out In their mothers' bosom.

13 How shall I console you? To what shall I liken you, O daughter of Jerusalem?

What shall I compare with you, that I may comfort you, O virgin daughter of Zion? For your ruin is spread wide as the sea; Who can heal you?

Summary

This passage offers a vivid and sorrowful portrayal of the prophet Jeremiah's anguish following the destruction of Jerusalem. It captures the emotional and physical toll that witnessing such devastation has taken on him. Jeremiah is depicted as deeply heartbroken—openly weeping and physically affected by the suffering around him. His grief is especially intense as he watches the most vulnerable, including children and infants, dying of hunger in the streets. These scenes overwhelm him with profound sadness and helplessness.

The text emphasizes the cries of the innocent, painting a picture of a desperate and broken population. Children beg their mothers for food and water, only to collapse and die in their arms. This heartbreaking imagery reveals not only the physical suffering caused by famine and war, but also the emotional torment endured by families. The mothers, unable to save their children, embody the depth of human vulnerability in the face of overwhelming catastrophe.

Jeremiah's lament reaches a point where words fail him. The destruction is so vast and painful that he cannot find a metaphor strong enough to describe it. He is left asking who might comfort Jerusalem or bring healing to its wounds. The devastation is not only physical—it is spiritual and communal. The city's identity, its covenant with God, and its sense of purpose have all been shattered. Jeremiah longs for restoration, yet feels the weight of hopelessness.

The Hebrew word translated as "heal" in this passage is *rapha*, which means to heal, repair, or make whole. In this context, *rapha* refers to more than physical recovery—it speaks to the full restoration of Israel. It includes the renewal of the people's spiritual identity, the mending of broken relationships, and the reestablishment of covenantal connection with God. The use of *rapha* underscores the hope that, even in the face of overwhelming loss, divine healing is still possible.

Ultimately, this passage reflects the tension between despair and hope, judgment and mercy. It affirms that while suffering may be great, God's compassion remains. Jeremiah's cry is not just one of grief—it is a plea for restoration. Through *rapha*, the text points to the enduring possibility of healing, reminding us that even in the darkest moments, renewal can come through divine grace.

Chapter 10
Heal in the book of Hosea

1. Hosea 5:11-13

11 Ephraim is oppressed and broken in judgment, Because he willingly walked by human precept.

12 Therefore I will be to Ephraim like a moth, And to the house of Judah like rottenness.

13 "When Ephraim saw his sickness, And Judah saw his wound, Then Ephraim went to Assyria And sent to King Jareb; Yet he cannot cure you, Nor heal you of your wound.

Summary

This passage from the prophetic book of Hosea delivers a serious message of divine judgment against the kingdoms of Israel and Judah—represented by Ephraim and the southern region. It addresses the spiritual decline of both nations, who have turned away from God and placed their trust in human strategies and foreign alliances instead of relying on divine guidance. Their abandonment of covenant faithfulness leads to unavoidable consequences.

God declares that He will be like a moth to Ephraim and like decay to Judah. These metaphors suggest a slow and subtle form of judgment. Rather than sudden destruction, the punishment unfolds gradually, weakening the nations from within. This quiet erosion reflects God's response not only to their idolatry but also to their refusal to seek restoration through repentance.

Instead of returning to God for healing, Israel and Judah look to external powers like Assyria, hoping that political alliances and military strength will save them. This misplaced trust reveals their spiritual blindness. The nations they turn to cannot heal their wounds or protect them from divine justice. Their efforts are in vain because the root of their suffering is not political—it is spiritual. Only God can address the true cause of their brokenness.

The Hebrew word translated as "heal" in this passage is *rapha*, which means to heal, repair, or make whole. In this context, *rapha* refers to the kind of restoration that only God can provide. It is not limited to physical recovery but includes spiritual renewal and the repair of the broken covenant relationship. The use of *rapha* emphasizes the depth of the damage and the need for divine intervention to restore what has been lost.

Ultimately, this passage serves as a strong reminder of the danger of turning away from God and the futility of seeking salvation apart from Him. It calls the people to repentance and highlights that true healing—*rapha*—comes only through returning to the

Lord. God alone can restore what has been damaged, renew what has been lost, and bring wholeness where there is brokenness. This message remains timeless: healing begins not with human solutions, but with humble surrender to the One who heals completely.

2. Hosea 6:1

Come, and let us return to the Lord; For He has torn, but He will heal us; He has stricken, but He will bind us up.

Summary

This passage from the book of Hosea offers a heartfelt call to repentance, urging the people of Israel to return to God after a time of spiritual separation. The prophet reminds them that the same God who has wounded them in judgment is also the one who desires to heal and restore. The imagery of tearing and wounding is not meant to portray cruelty, but to reflect the serious consequences of rebellion and the depth of divine discipline. Yet, this is immediately followed by a promise of healing—a clear expression of God's enduring mercy.

The Hebrew word translated as "heal" in this passage is *rapha*, which carries a rich and layered meaning. It refers not only to physical recovery but also to repair, restoration, and making whole. In this context, *rapha* speaks to the full scope of divine healing. Hosea's message reveals that God's restoration is holistic: He can mend the broken body, renew the wounded soul, restore fractured families, and rebuild a nation shaken by sin. His healing reaches into every area touched by chaos and devastation, offering renewal to those who turn back to Him.

This passage highlights the compassionate nature of God. He is not distant or indifferent to suffering; rather, He stands ready to forgive and restore those who come to Him in humility. Whether the damage is personal, relational, or national, the process of healing begins with repentance. Hosea outlines two essential conditions for restoration: first, the recognition of brokenness—whether in an individual, a household, or a nation; and second, a sincere return to God, even while still in the midst of that brokenness. God does not require perfection, but a heart willing to seek Him.

Ultimately, Hosea's message is one of hope. It affirms that no situation is beyond the reach of divine healing, and that God's mercy always exceeds His judgment. Through repentance and faith, healing is not only possible—it is assured. The use of *rapha* in this passage reminds us that God's restoration is complete, reaching into every layer of human need. It is a promise that brokenness is not the end, and that renewal awaits those who return to the Lord with open hearts.

3. Hosea 14:1-4

1 O Israel, return to the Lord your God, For you have stumbled because of your iniquity;

2 Take words with you, And return to the Lord. Say to Him, "Take away all iniquity; Receive us graciously, For we will offer the sacrifices of our lips.

3 Assyria shall not save us, We will not ride on horses, Nor will we say anymore to the work of our hands, 'You are our gods.' For in You the fatherless finds mercy."

4 I will heal their backsliding, I will love them freely, For My anger has turned away from him.

Summary

This passage from the book of Hosea offers a heartfelt and urgent call to repentance. The prophet pleads with the people of Israel to turn away from their sins and return to the Lord. Hosea does not speak in vague terms—he provides a clear example of what true repentance should sound like: an honest confession of wrongdoing and a humble request for mercy. He urges the people to pray, "Forgive all iniquity, receive us graciously, for we will offer the sacrifices of our lips." This statement marks a significant shift from empty ritual to sincere worship, where words of praise and repentance replace outward offerings.

Hosea also challenges the people to abandon their misplaced trust in political powers and military strength. He makes it clear that salvation will not come from Assyria, from war horses, or from idols made by human hands. These false sources of security cannot save. True deliverance comes only from God, who shows compassion even to those who are abandoned and without support.

In response to this anticipated return, God offers a powerful promise. He declares that He will heal their unfaithfulness, love them freely, and turn away His anger. These assurances reveal the depth of God's mercy and His desire to restore those who come back to Him with sincerity. The healing God offers is not just physical—it is spiritual and relational. It addresses the broken covenant, the wounded hearts, and the fractured identity of a people who have strayed.

The Hebrew word translated as "heal" is *rapha*, which means to heal, repair, or make whole. In this context, *rapha* speaks to God's intention to restore what has been damaged by sin. It includes forgiveness, renewal, and the rebuilding of a loving relationship between God and His people. This healing is complete—it touches every part of life, from the individual heart to the national identity.

Ultimately, this passage highlights the power of repentance and the limitless grace of God. It reminds us that no matter how far we have wandered, restoration is always possible. God does not wait with condemnation, but with compassion. Through *rapha*, He offers healing that is deep, lasting, and full of hope for all who return to Him with open hearts.

Chapter 11
Heal in the book of Zechariah

1. Zechariah 11:15-17

15 And the Lord said to me, "Next, take for yourself the implements of a foolish shepherd.

16 For indeed I will raise up a shepherd in the land who will not care for those who are cut off, nor seek the young, nor heal those that are broken, nor feed those that still stand. But he will eat the flesh of the fat and tear their hooves in pieces.

17 "Woe to the worthless shepherd, Who leaves the flock! A sword shall be against his arm And against his right eye; His arm shall completely wither, And his right eye shall be totally blinded."

Summary

This passage from the book of Zechariah offers a sobering depiction of divine judgment against corrupt and negligent spiritual leaders. God instructs the prophet Zechariah to take on the symbolic role of a "foolish shepherd," representing those who have failed in their sacred responsibility to care for the people entrusted to them. These leaders are marked by their disregard for the weak, their neglect of the sick, and their unwillingness to protect the vulnerable. Instead of serving the flock, they exploit it for personal gain, abandoning the principles of compassion, justice, and faithful stewardship.

Through this prophetic act, God exposes the moral and spiritual failures of such leadership and issues a clear warning: their strength will be broken, and their vision will be darkened. This judgment reflects how seriously God views leadership, especially within the spiritual community. Those who misuse their authority and betray their calling will face divine accountability. The image of the shepherd—typically associated with care, guidance, and protection—is here reversed to emphasize the consequences of betrayal and abuse.

This passage affirms that God is neither blind to injustice nor indifferent to the suffering of His people. He sees the damage caused by irresponsible leaders and promises that such harm will not go unanswered. It serves as a powerful reminder that leadership is not a privilege for self-interest but a sacred trust. Those who lead are accountable to God for the well-being of those they serve.

The Hebrew word translated as "heal" in this passage is *rapha*, meaning to heal, repair, or make whole. In this context, *rapha* represents the restoration that the foolish shepherd fails to provide. The absence of healing highlights the leader's failure, while the word itself points to what true leadership should offer: the renewal and care of the community. Healing, in its fullest sense, is not just physical—it is spiritual, emotional, and relational. It involves restoring dignity, rebuilding trust, and nurturing wholeness.

Ultimately, this passage calls for integrity, compassion, and accountability in leadership. It assures that divine justice will prevail and that God will not overlook the suffering of His people. Through the lens of *rapha*, we see that true leadership is marked by the ability to restore, to protect, and to serve with humility and grace.

PART 2

HEALED IN THE OLD TESTAMENT

Chapter 12
Healed in the book of Genesis

1. Genesis 20:17-18

17 So Abraham prayed to God; and God healed Abimelech, his wife, and his female servants. Then they bore children;

18 for the Lord had closed up all the wombs of the house of Abimelech because of Sarah, Abraham's wife.

Summary

In this passage from the Book of Genesis, traditionally attributed to Moses, we encounter a significant moment in Abraham's journey through the land of Gerar. Upon arriving, Abraham faces a sensitive challenge involving his wife, Sarah. Because of her miraculous rejuvenation—understood as part of God's covenantal promise (See Genesis 18:10-12)—Abraham fears that her beauty might attract unwanted attention and endanger both of them. To protect her, he presents Sarah as his sister, a decision that, while strategic, leads to unintended consequences.

King Abimelech, unaware of the true nature of their relationship, sends for Sarah and brings her into his palace. This action triggers divine intervention. God appears to Abimelech in a dream, warning him of the serious implications of his actions. He reveals that Abimelech's household has been afflicted with barrenness—a direct result of taking Sarah. God then instructs the king to return Sarah to Abraham and informs him that Abraham is a prophet. Importantly, God tells Abimelech to seek Abraham's prayer, promising that through this intercession, healing and restoration will come to his household.

Abimelech obeys, returning Sarah and requesting Abraham's prayer. In response, Abraham intercedes, and God heals Abimelech and his household, restoring their ability to bear children and lifting the divine judgment. This episode highlights several key theological themes: God's sovereignty over human affairs, the sacredness of covenant relationships, and the power of intercessory prayer. It also affirms Sarah's protected role in God's redemptive plan, reinforcing her significance in the fulfillment of the promise to Abraham.

The Hebrew word translated as "heal" in this passage is *rapha*, a term rich in meaning. While it often refers to physical healing, *rapha* also conveys the broader idea of restoration and renewal. It implies repairing or bringing something back to its original, intended state—whether that be a person's health, a family's well-being, or a spiritual condition. In this context, *rapha* signifies more than the reversal of barrenness;

it represents the reestablishment of divine order and blessing within Abimelech's household.

Ultimately, this passage affirms that healing is not merely a physical act but a spiritual restoration initiated by God. It underscores the importance of prophetic intercession and the faithfulness of God to protect those chosen to fulfill His covenant. Through *rapha*, we see that divine healing is both a sign of mercy and a reaffirmation of God's commitment to His promises.

Chapter 13
Healed in the book of Exodus

1. Exodus 21:18-19

18 "If men contend with each other, and one strikes the other with a stone or with his fist, and he does not die but is confined to his bed,

19 if he rises again and walks about outside with his staff, then he who struck him shall be acquitted. He shall only pay for the loss of his time, and shall provide for him to be thoroughly healed.

Summary

In this passage from the Book of Exodus, Moses presents a legal instruction to the people of Israel that addresses personal injury and the responsibilities that follow. He describes a situation in which two individuals become involved in a physical conflict, and one man strikes the other—either with his hand or an object like a stone—resulting in the victim being injured and unable to work. Although the injury is not fatal and does not warrant capital punishment, the aggressor is still held accountable for the harm caused.

The law requires the offender to compensate the injured person for any lost time and to provide for his care until he has fully recovered. This legal requirement reflects a key principle in biblical justice: the focus is not on punishment alone, but on restoration. The goal is to ensure that the injured person's dignity, livelihood, and well-being are protected. This approach promotes a sense of social responsibility, where those who cause harm are expected to take part in the healing process of those they have wronged.

This passage also reveals a deeper theological message. It shows God's concern for human life and well-being, emphasizing that justice includes care and compassion. The emphasis on recovery and restoration aligns with broader biblical themes, particularly the healing nature of God's character.

The Hebrew word translated as "healed" in this context is *rapha*, a word rich in meaning. While *rapha* often refers to physical healing, it also carries the broader sense of restoration and renewal. It implies bringing something back to its original, whole, and functional state—whether that be a person's health, a relationship, or the social order. In this legal setting, *rapha* points not only to the physical recovery of the injured person but also to the restoration of justice and balance within the community.

This vision of healing is holistic. It includes physical care, emotional support, and social responsibility. The law does not simply aim to resolve conflict but to restore what was broken. In doing so, it reflects the covenant values of compassion, accountability, and care that are central to Israel's identity as God's people.

Ultimately, this passage affirms that healing—*rapha*—is not just a personal matter but a communal responsibility. It calls individuals to participate in the restoration of others, echoing the divine desire to bring wholeness and justice to every part of life.

Chapter 14
Healed in the book of Leviticus

1. Leviticus 13:18-23

18 "If the body develops a boil in the skin, and it is healed,

19 and in the place of the boil there comes a white swelling or a bright spot, reddish-white, then it shall be shown to the priest;

20 and if, when the priest sees it, it indeed appears deeper than the skin, and its hair has turned white, the priest shall pronounce him unclean. It is a leprous sore which has broken out of the boil.

21 But if the priest examines it, and indeed there are no white hairs in it, and it is not deeper than the skin, but has faded, then the priest shall isolate him seven days;

22 and if it should at all spread over the skin, then the priest shall pronounce him unclean. It is a leprous sore.

23 But if the bright spot stays in one place, and has not spread, it is the scar of the boil; and the priest shall pronounce him clean.

Summary

In this passage from the Book of Leviticus, Moses outlines a detailed system for identifying and managing skin conditions, especially those resembling leprosy. These instructions serve both medical and spiritual purposes, emphasizing the importance of ritual purity, public health, and divine order within the community of Israel.

The process begins when someone who has recovered from a boil develops a white swelling or reddish spot. Such symptoms must be examined by a priest, who acts not only as a spiritual leader but also as a health official. The priest's role is to assess whether the condition is leprous, which would render the individual ritually unclean and require isolation from the community.

Moses provides clear criteria to help distinguish leprosy from other skin issues. If the sore appears deeper than the skin and the hairs within it have turned white, the priest is to declare the person unclean. If the sore is more superficial, lacks white hairs, and appears pale, the individual is to be quarantined for seven days. After this period, if the sore has spread, the diagnosis confirms leprosy. If it remains unchanged and does not spread, the person is declared clean and allowed to rejoin the community.

This passage highlights the priest's dual responsibility: diagnosing illness and overseeing the healing process. Their duties include enforcing isolation to prevent the spread of disease and confirming recovery before reintegration. These procedures reflect a broader concern for both physical health and spiritual integrity, ensuring that the community remains whole and protected.

The concept of healing in this context is deeply connected to the Hebrew word *rapha*, which carries rich meaning. While *rapha* often refers to physical healing, it also includes the idea of restoration—bringing someone or something back to its original, functional state. It reflects God's power not only to cure illness but also to renew relationships, restore dignity, and reestablish harmony within the community.

In this passage, *rapha* is not limited to the physical recovery of the individual. It symbolizes the broader divine intention to restore order and well-being. Healing is seen as a sacred act, involving both human responsibility and divine compassion. The priest's role in this process reflects God's covenantal care, ensuring that those who suffer are not forgotten but are guided toward restoration.

Ultimately, this passage affirms that healing—*rapha*—is a holistic process. It involves physical recovery, spiritual renewal, and social reintegration, all grounded in God's faithful concern for His people.

2. Leviticus 13:34-37

34 On the seventh day the priest shall examine the scale; and indeed if the scale has not spread over the

skin, and does not appear deeper than the skin, then the priest shall pronounce him clean. He shall wash his clothes and be clean.

35 But if the scale should at all spread over the skin after his cleansing,

36 then the priest shall examine him; and indeed if the scale has spread over the skin, the priest need not seek for yellow hair. He is unclean.

37 But if the scale appears to be at a standstill, and there is black hair grown up in it, the scale has healed. He is clean, and the priest shall pronounce him clean.

Summary

In this passage from the Book of Leviticus, Moses provides detailed instructions to the priests regarding the identification and management of infectious skin conditions affecting the scalp and beard. These regulations form part of a broader framework designed to preserve both public health and ritual purity within the community of Israel. The procedures reflect a careful balance between medical observation and spiritual responsibility, emphasizing the importance of maintaining communal well-being.

The text outlines a structured process for diagnosing conditions resembling leprosy, particularly those similar to ringworm, which was considered a form of leprosy when it appeared on the head or beard. When an individual presents with a sore in these areas, the priest is tasked with examining the lesion closely. If the sore appears deeper than the surface of the skin and contains fine, yellowish hairs, the priest must declare the person unclean, confirming the presence of a contagious condition.

If the sore is not deep and lacks black hairs, the individual is placed in isolation for seven days. After this initial period, the priest reexamines the area. If the condition has not spread, shows no yellowish hairs, and remains superficial, the person must shave their head—excluding the infected area—and undergo a second seven-day quarantine. At the end of this phase, the priest conducts another assessment. If the lesion remains unchanged and shallow, the person is declared clean. They are then instructed to wash their garments as part of the purification process and present themselves for final confirmation.

However, if the condition worsens after purification, the priest does not need to look for yellow hairs; the individual is automatically considered unclean. On the other hand, if the lesion remains stable and black hairs begin to grow, this is recognized as a sign of healing. The priest then confirms the person's recovery, allowing them to rejoin the community.

This passage highlights the priest's essential role in maintaining both physical health and ritual integrity. The procedures demonstrate a thoughtful approach to disease control, incorporating isolation, careful observation, and gradual reintegration. They reflect a deep concern for the individual's well-being and the health of the wider community.

The Hebrew word translated as "healed" in this context is *rapha*, which means to heal or restore. More than physical recovery, *rapha* conveys the idea of renewal—bringing someone or something back to its intended, whole state. In this passage, healing is not simply the absence of illness but the restoration of full participation in the covenant community, affirming God's desire for wholeness in both body and spirit.

3. Leviticus 14:1-4

1 Then the Lord spoke to Moses, saying,

2 "This shall be the law of the leper for the day of his cleansing: He shall be brought to the priest.

3 And the priest shall go out of the camp, and the priest shall examine him; and indeed, if the leprosy is healed in the leper,

4 then the priest shall command to take for him who is to be cleansed two living and clean birds, cedar wood, scarlet, and hyssop.

Summary

In this passage from the Book of Leviticus, God gives Moses detailed instructions for the ritual cleansing of individuals who have recovered from leprosy. These laws reflect the deep connection between physical healing, spiritual renewal, and social restoration in ancient Israelite life. According to the law, once a person shows signs of recovery, they must be brought to a priest for examination. This takes place outside the camp, symbolizing the separation required during their time of impurity.

If the priest confirms that the person has been healed, a specific purification ritual begins. This ceremony involves several symbolic items: two live, ceremonially clean birds, cedar wood, scarlet yarn, and hyssop. Each element carries spiritual meaning. One bird is sacrificed, while the other is released, representing the person's return to life and freedom. Cedar wood, known for its strength and fragrance, symbolizes purification and endurance. Scarlet yarn points to sacrifice and redemption, and hyssop, often used in cleansing rites, highlights the theme of spiritual renewal.

The priest plays a vital role in this process—not only as a religious leader but also as a caretaker of public health and ritual order. He is responsible for confirming the person's physical recovery and guiding them through the steps that restore their place in the community. This ensures that healing is not limited to the body but includes the person's spiritual and social reintegration.

The Hebrew word translated as "healed" in this passage is *rapha*, a word rich in meaning. While it often refers to physical healing, *rapha* also conveys the idea of restoration—bringing something back to its original, whole, and functional state. In this context, *rapha* reflects more than the end of illness; it signifies the full restoration of the individual's dignity, identity, and place within the covenant community.

This passage affirms that healing in the biblical tradition is a holistic process. It involves more than curing disease—it includes renewing the spirit, restoring relationships, and reestablishing one's role in the community. The ritual reflects God's compassionate desire not only to heal but to make whole. Through the priest's careful attention and the symbolic acts of the ritual, the person is welcomed back into fellowship, fully restored in body, soul, and social standing.

Ultimately, this text reveals that *rapha* is not just about physical recovery—it is about the complete renewal of life, guided by divine mercy and covenantal care.

4. Leviticus 14:46-48

46 Moreover he who goes into the house at all while it is shut up shall be unclean until evening.

47 And he who lies down in the house shall wash his clothes, and he who eats in the house shall wash his clothes.

48 "But if the priest comes in and examines it, and indeed the plague has not spread in the house after the house was plastered, then the priest shall pronounce the house clean, because the plague is healed.

Summary

In this passage from the Book of Leviticus, God gives Moses detailed instructions for identifying and managing houses suspected of being contaminated with a form of leprosy. These guidelines reflect a divine concern for both physical cleanliness and communal well-being, emphasizing the importance of hygiene, containment, and spiritual integrity within the covenant community.

When a house shows signs of possible infestation—specifically greenish or reddish streaks embedded in its walls—the owner must report the issue to a priest. Before inspecting the house, the priest orders it to be emptied to prevent the contents from becoming defiled if the house is later declared unclean. Upon examination, if the discoloration appears to penetrate the surface of the walls, the priest seals the house for seven days, prohibiting entry during this quarantine period.

After the seven days, the priest returns to reassess the condition. If the discoloration has spread, he orders the removal of the affected stones, which are to be discarded in a designated unclean area outside the city. New stones are then installed, and the house is replastered. A follow-up inspection determines whether the infestation has returned. If it has, the house is declared irreparably defiled and must be demolished. Anyone who enters the house during this time becomes ceremonially unclean until evening and must wash their garments.

However, if the discoloration does not reappear after the repairs, the priest declares the house clean, signifying that the affliction has been resolved. This process ensures not only the physical safety of the inhabitants but also the spiritual purity of the community. It reflects a holistic approach to restoration—one that integrates health, ritual observance, and social responsibility.

The Hebrew word translated as "healed" in this context is *rapha*, a term that goes beyond physical recovery. While *rapha* commonly refers to healing or curing, it also conveys the idea of restoration—bringing something back to its original, functional state. In this passage, *rapha* applies not only to individuals but also to dwellings and environments, highlighting God's power to renew and purify all aspects of life.

Ultimately, this text affirms the sacred responsibility of maintaining health, order, and holiness within the covenant community. It underscores the priest's role as both guardian of public well-being and mediator of divine standards. Through the lens of *rapha*, healing is understood as a comprehensive act of renewal—restoring what was broken and reaffirming God's presence among His people.

Chapter 15
Healed in the book of Deuteronomy

1. Deuteronomy 28:25-27

25 "The Lord will cause you to be defeated before your enemies; you shall go out one way against them and flee seven ways before them; and you shall become troublesome to all the kingdoms of the earth.

26 Your carcasses shall be food for all the birds of the air and the beasts of the earth, and no one shall frighten them away.

27 The Lord will strike you with the boils of Egypt, with tumors, with the scab, and with the itch, from which you cannot be healed.

Summary

In this passage from the Book of Deuteronomy, God presents a solemn warning to the people of Israel about the consequences of breaking His commandments. After outlining the blessings that come with obedience—such as prosperity, protection, and divine favor—God turns to the serious outcomes of disobedience. These warnings are direct and intense, emphasizing the weight of turning away from the covenant.

Among the consequences described are military defeat and national dispersion. The people will be forced to flee from their enemies, becoming scattered and vulnerable. Their suffering will be so severe that other nations will look on with shock and fear. The text also speaks of death in battle, and the absence of burial rites—a loss of dignity that leaves bodies exposed to birds and wild animals. These images reflect not only physical pain but also a sense of spiritual abandonment.

The passage goes further to describe bodily afflictions—painful and incurable diseases, including those linked to the plagues of Egypt. Conditions such as hemorrhoids, scabies, and ringworm are mentioned, highlighting the persistent and humiliating nature of these illnesses. These are not just physical ailments; they symbolize divine judgment and the withdrawal of God's protective presence.

This section of Deuteronomy serves as a powerful reminder of the covenant between God and His people. Disobedience breaks that relationship, leading to both physical suffering and spiritual isolation. Without God's protection, the people are left exposed to shame, hardship, and disorder.

The Hebrew word translated as "healed" in this context is *rapha*, a term rich in meaning. While *rapha* often refers to physical healing, it also conveys the idea of restoration—repairing or renewing something to its original, whole, and functional state. In Scripture, *rapha* frequently signifies complete healing, including emotional and spiritual renewal.

In contrast to the incurable diseases described in this passage, *rapha* represents God's power to restore what has been broken. Its absence here underscores the seriousness of divine judgment and the importance of remaining faithful to the covenant. Healing is not automatic—it is tied to obedience, humility, and relationship with God.

Ultimately, this passage affirms that obedience is more than a moral duty—it is the path to wholeness, protection, and divine favor. Through *rapha*, God offers not just relief from suffering but full restoration, reminding His people that healing flows from covenantal faithfulness.

2. Deuteronomy 28:33-35

33 A nation whom you have not known shall eat the fruit of your land and the produce of your labor, and you shall be only oppressed and crushed continually.

34 So you shall be driven mad because of the sight which your eyes see.

35 The Lord will strike you in the knees and on the legs with severe boils which cannot be healed, and from the sole of your foot to the top of your head.

Summary

In this passage from the Book of Deuteronomy, God continues to warn the people of Israel about the serious consequences of disobedience. These warnings follow a detailed list of blessings tied to obedience and serve as a solemn reminder of the covenant between God and His people. The text emphasizes that turning away from God's commandments leads not only to loss but to deep suffering across every part of life.

Among the curses described is the loss of agricultural and economic prosperity. The hard work of the Israelites—whether in farming or other labor—will benefit foreign nations instead of themselves. This loss of productivity and control reflects a withdrawal of divine favor and signals a weakening of national strength and identity.

The passage also warns of harsh oppression by foreign powers. The Israelites will be overwhelmed by external domination, and the constant exposure to suffering will lead to emotional and mental distress. The text paints a vivid picture of despair, where the burden of affliction becomes so great that it drives people to madness.

One of the most striking aspects of this warning is the physical suffering that results from disobedience. God will allow incurable boils to appear on the knees and legs of the people, symbolizing pain, immobility, and helplessness. These afflictions are described as irreversible, underscoring the seriousness of divine judgment and the absence of healing outside the boundaries of covenant faithfulness.

This passage reveals the layered nature of divine retribution—economic hardship, social collapse, psychological torment, and physical pain. It serves as a powerful caution against rejecting God's instructions and highlights the devastating impact of breaking covenantal trust.

The Hebrew word translated as "healed" in this context is *rapha*, a term rich in theological meaning. While *rapha* often refers to physical healing, it also conveys the idea of restoration—repairing or renewing something to its original, whole, and functional state. In Scripture, *rapha* frequently points to holistic healing, encompassing body, spirit, and community.

In contrast to the incurable conditions described in this passage, *rapha* represents God's power to restore what is broken. Its absence here emphasizes the seriousness of disobedience and the need to remain within God's covenant to receive healing and renewal.

Ultimately, this passage affirms that obedience is not just a moral duty—it is the path to wholeness. Through *rapha*, God offers restoration, but only to those who walk in faithfulness and trust.

Chapter 16
Healed in the book of Samuel

1. 1 Samuel 6:1-3

1 Now the ark of the Lord was in the country of the Philistines seven months.

2 And the Philistines called for the priests and the diviners, saying, "What shall we do with the ark of the Lord? Tell us how we should send it to its place."

3 So they said, "If you send away the ark of the God of Israel, do not send it empty; but by all means return it to Him with a trespass offering. Then you will be healed, and it will be known to you why His hand is not removed from you."

Summary

This passage from the First Book of Samuel recounts a pivotal moment in Israel's history involving the Ark of the Covenant. Due to the disobedience of the people and the irreverent behavior of Eli's sons—who failed to honor the sacredness of the Ark—God allowed it to be captured by the Philistines. This event marked a moment of divine judgment and signaled the withdrawal of God's protective presence from Israel.

The Philistines held the Ark for seven months, during which their cities were struck by devastation, disease, and plagues. These afflictions were understood as direct consequences of possessing the Ark without reverence or recognition of its holiness. Realizing the severity of their suffering and attributing it to the displeasure of the God of Israel, the Philistines decided to return the Ark.

To ensure they acted appropriately, they consulted their priests and diviners for guidance. These religious advisors instructed them to send the Ark back with a guilt offering—golden images representing the plagues that had afflicted them. This offering was meant to acknowledge their wrongdoing, express repentance, and seek relief from their suffering. It was a symbolic act of submission to divine authority and a plea for restoration.

This narrative highlights the Philistines' recognition of the power and holiness of the God of Israel. Though they were not part of the covenant community, they responded with humility and reverence. Their actions reflect a broader theological truth: that divine judgment is not limited to Israel, and that healing is available to all who approach God with sincerity and repentance.

The Hebrew word translated as "healed" in this context is *rapha*, a term that carries deep theological meaning. While it often refers to physical healing, *rapha* also encompasses restoration—bringing something back to its original, whole, and functional state. In this passage, healing is not simply the end of disease; it represents the renewal of order, the restoration of reverence, and the return of divine favor.

Ultimately, this account affirms the seriousness of approaching what is sacred with respect and the transformative power of repentance. Through the lens of *rapha*, healing is understood as a divine act that restores not only health but also relationship, dignity, and peace. The Philistines' experience serves as a reminder that God's mercy is available—even to outsiders—when approached with humility and a desire for restoration.

Chapter 17
Healed in the book of Kings

1. 2 Kings 2:19-22

19 Then the men of the city said to Elisha, "Please notice, the situation of this city is pleasant, as my lord sees; but the water is bad, and the ground barren."

20 And he said, "Bring me a new bowl, and put salt in it." So they brought it to him.

21 Then he went out to the source of the water, and cast in the salt there, and said, "Thus says the Lord: 'I have healed this water; from it there shall be no more death or barrenness.' "

22 So the water remains healed to this day, according to the word of Elisha which he spoke.

Summary

This passage recounts a remarkable moment in the ministry of the prophet Elisha, shortly after he succeeded Elijah. During a visit to the city of Jericho, the local residents approached Elisha with a serious concern: the city's spring produced harmful water, which caused widespread unfruitfulness and hardship. Although Jericho was well situated geographically, the land could not thrive because its water source was tainted. The people were living in a place of promise, yet the environment around them was broken and unable to support life.

In response, Elisha asked for a new bowl filled with salt. He went to the spring and, in a symbolic act, threw the salt into the water. Then he declared, "This is what the Lord says: I have healed this water. Never again will it cause death or make the land unproductive." From that moment, the water was restored, and the land began to flourish again.

This account reveals more than just a miracle—it shows the power of divine healing reaching beyond human bodies to the natural world. The phrase "I have healed this water" reflects a broader understanding of what it means for something to be "sick." In Scripture, when something no longer functions according to its God-given purpose—whether a person, a community, or even a spring—it is seen as needing healing. Water is meant to give life. When it brings harm instead, it is considered broken and in need of restoration.

This story invites us to reflect on the nature of healing in the Bible. The Hebrew word *rapha*, often translated as "to heal," carries a rich meaning. It includes not only physical recovery but also the idea of repairing, renewing, and restoring something to its proper and life-giving state. In this passage, *rapha* is not limited to human health—it extends to the environment, showing that God's healing power touches all of creation.

Elisha's act, and the Lord's declaration, demonstrate that healing is part of God's desire to restore wholeness wherever there is brokenness. Whether in a body, a relationship, or a landscape, God's power to *rapha*—to heal and make whole—is active and available. This story reminds us that healing is not only about relief from suffering but about restoring things to their true purpose: to give life, to bless, and to reflect the goodness of God.

2. 2 Kings 8:28-29 (KJV)

28 And he went with Joram the son of Ahab to the war against Hazael king of Syria in Ramoth Gilead; and the Syrians wounded Joram.

29 And king Joram went back to be healed in Jezreel of the wounds which the Syrians had given him at Ramah, when he fought against Hazael king of Syria. And Ahaziah the son of Jehoram king of Judah went down to see Joram the son of Ahab in Jezreel, because he was sick.

Summary

This passage offers a glimpse into the complex political and spiritual dynamics of the divided monarchy period in ancient Israel. It centers on Jehoram, son of Ahab and king of Israel, during his military campaign against the king of Syria at Ramoth-Gilead. Jehoram is accompanied by King Ahaziah of Judah, whose alliance with Israel was strengthened through marriage into Ahab's family. This partnership reflects the intricate and often fragile relationships between the northern kingdom of Israel and the southern kingdom of Judah.

During the battle, Jehoram is wounded by Syrian forces and must retreat from the front lines. He returns to Jezreel to recover from his injuries. While he is healing, King Ahaziah visits him, reinforcing the political and familial bonds between the two rulers. Their meeting highlights the shared interests and mutual dependencies that shaped the leadership landscape of the time. It also reveals how personal health and national stability were closely linked—when a king was wounded, the entire kingdom felt the impact.

Beyond the political and military details, this passage introduces a deeper theme: healing and restoration. The Hebrew word used for "healed" is *rapha*, which traditionally refers to physical recovery. However, *rapha* carries a broader meaning. It speaks of restoration, renewal, and the return to proper function. In this context, Jehoram's healing is not only about his physical condition—it symbolizes the possibility of renewal in leadership, alliance, and spiritual direction.

The use of *rapha* invites reflection on how healing in the Bible often goes beyond the body. It can represent the restoration of relationships, the mending of political fractures, or the renewal of divine favor. Jehoram's recovery, though personal, hints at the potential for broader restoration—within his kingdom, his alliances, and perhaps even his relationship with God.

This episode also subtly points to divine providence. While the text does not describe a miraculous healing, the process of recovery itself is seen as part of God's sustaining work. The presence of *rapha* reminds us that healing—whether slow or sudden—is a sign of God's desire to restore what is broken.

Ultimately, this passage illustrates the interconnectedness of health, leadership, and divine purpose. It shows that healing is not just a private matter—it has public and spiritual significance. Through the lens of *rapha*, we see that restoration is always possible, and that God's healing touch can reach into every corner of life, from the battlefield to the throne.

3. 2 Kings 9:14-16 (KJV)

14 So Jehu the son of Jehoshaphat the son of Nimshi conspired against Joram. (Now Joram had kept Ramothgilead, he and all Israel, because of Hazael king of Syria.

15 But king Joram was returned to be healed in Jezreel of the wounds which the Syrians had given him, when he fought with Hazael king of Syria.) And Jehu said, If it be your minds, then let none go forth nor escape out of the city to go to tell it in Jezreel.

16 So Jehu rode in a chariot, and went to Jezreel; for Joram lay there. And Ahaziah king of Judah was come down to see Joram.

Summary

This passage recounts the dramatic rise of Jehu, son of Jehoshaphat and Nimshi, a military commander in Israel whose unexpected ascent to kingship was foretold by the prophet Elisha. Acting on this divine message, Jehu was declared king by the officers serving under King Jehoram, the reigning monarch of Israel. At the time, Jehoram was recovering in Jezreel from injuries sustained during a battle at Ramoth-Gilead against Hazael, king of Syria.

Recognizing the strategic opportunity, Jehu launched a swift and calculated plan. He ordered his men to block any escape from Ramoth-Gilead, ensuring that news of his anointing would not spread prematurely. He then traveled to Jezreel, where he carried out a series of bold and decisive actions. Jehu killed Jehoram, king of Israel; Ahaziah, king of Judah; and Jezebel, the powerful widow of Ahab. These acts fulfilled the prophetic judgments previously spoken by Elijah and Elisha, marking a moment of divine reckoning against the house of Ahab.

This passage represents a turning point in Israel's political and spiritual history. Jehu's rise to power brought significant changes to national leadership and religious direction. Though his actions were violent, they were understood within the framework of divine justice and covenantal accountability. The prophets had warned of judgment, and Jehu's mission was seen as the fulfillment of those warnings.

The theme of healing is subtly woven into this narrative through the Hebrew word *rapha*, often translated as "healed" or "restored." While *rapha* typically refers to physical healing, its deeper meaning includes the ideas of rehabilitation, renewal, and returning something to its proper and functional state. In this context, Jehu's rise can be viewed as a form of divine *rapha*—a restoration of Israel's leadership and spiritual direction after a period of corruption and decline.

Jehu's actions, though forceful, were part of a larger process of renewal. The removal of leaders who had led the people astray was not just political—it was spiritual. It was an effort to cleanse the nation and restore its covenant with God. Through the lens of *rapha*, this story becomes more than a tale of power—it becomes a testimony to God's commitment to heal what is broken, even in the realm of governance and national identity.

In this way, the passage invites us to see divine healing not only in personal terms but also in the restoration of communities, systems, and spiritual integrity.

Chapter 18
Healed in the book of Chronicles

1. 2 Chronicles 22:3-6 (KJV)

3 He also walked in the ways of the house of Ahab: for his mother was his counsellor to do wickedly.

4 Wherefore he did evil in the sight of the Lord like the house of Ahab: for they were his counsellors after the death of his father to his destruction.

5 He walked also after their counsel, and went with Jehoram the son of Ahab king of Israel to war against Hazael king of Syria at Ramothgilead: and the Syrians smote Joram.

6 And he returned to be healed in Jezreel because of the wounds which were given him at Ramah, when he fought with Hazael king of Syria. And Azariah the son of Jehoram king of Judah went down to see Jehoram the son of Ahab at Jezreel, because he was sick.

Summary

Following the death of Jehoram, king of Judah, his youngest son Ahaziah assumed the throne. His reign, however, was short and troubled, marked by poor decisions and spiritual compromise. Much of this was due to the influence of his mother, Athaliah, who came from the house of Ahab—a family known for leading Israel into idolatry and rebellion against God. Under her guidance, Ahaziah followed the same corrupt path, surrounding himself with advisors from Ahab's lineage and adopting practices that were offensive to the Lord.

Ahaziah's alliance with Jehoram, king of Israel and son of Ahab, further deepened his involvement in a legacy of disobedience. Together, they launched a military campaign against Hazael, king of Syria, at Ramoth-Gilead. The battle ended in disaster. Jehoram was seriously wounded and withdrew to Jezreel to recover. Ahaziah, showing loyalty, went to visit him. This act of solidarity, however, led to both their deaths. Jehu, a military commander anointed by God to bring judgment and reform, assassinated them as part of a divine mission to purge Israel of its corrupt leadership.

This passage highlights the dangers of ungodly alliances and the consequences of leadership shaped by unfaithful counsel. Ahaziah's downfall was not simply a result of military failure—it was rooted in spiritual compromise. His choices led him away from covenant faithfulness and into a path of destruction. The story serves as a warning about the influence of relationships and the importance of aligning leadership with God's will.

The Hebrew word often translated as "healed" in this context is *rapha*. While *rapha* can refer to physical healing, its deeper meaning includes restoration, renewal, and returning something to its proper and intended state. In contrast to the irreversible fate of Ahaziah and Jehoram, *rapha* represents God's ability to repair what has been broken—whether in a person, a nation, or a system of leadership.

This passage, therefore, is not only a record of political events but a spiritual lesson. It reminds us that healing—true *rapha*—comes through repentance, obedience, and alignment with God's purposes. While Ahaziah's story ends in judgment, the broader biblical message affirms that restoration is always possible when leaders and people turn back to God. *Rapha* is a promise of hope, showing that even in times of failure, God's desire is to heal and renew.

2. 2 Chronicles 30:17-20

17 For there were many in the assembly who had not sanctified themselves; therefore the Levites had charge of the slaughter of the Passover lambs for everyone who was not clean, to sanctify them to the Lord.

18 For a multitude of the people, many from Ephraim, Manasseh, Issachar, and Zebulun, had not cleansed themselves, yet they ate the Passover contrary to what was written. But Hezekiah prayed for them, saying, "May the good Lord provide atonement for everyone

19 who prepares his heart to seek God, the Lord God of his fathers, though he is not cleansed according to the purification of the sanctuary."

20 And the Lord listened to Hezekiah and healed the people.

Summary

This passage describes King Hezekiah's sincere efforts to restore the celebration of Passover across Israel after a long period of spiritual neglect. Following the cleansing and rededication of the Temple, Hezekiah called the nation back to covenant worship. His plan was thorough and intentional: he gathered the priests and Levites, instructed them to purify themselves and the Temple, and offered sin offerings on behalf of the kingdom. With the support of his leaders and the assembly, he chose a date for the Passover and sent messengers throughout the land, inviting all the tribes to come to Jerusalem and take part in the sacred feast.

Although some people mocked the invitation and refused to participate, many responded with sincerity. Delegations from tribes such as Ephraim, Manasseh, Issachar, and Zebulun traveled to Jerusalem. However, some of them joined the celebration without completing the required purification rituals. Seeing their genuine desire to seek God, Hezekiah prayed for them, saying, "May the good Lord pardon everyone who sets his heart to seek God...even if he is not cleansed according to the rules of the sanctuary." God heard Hezekiah's prayer and healed the people.

The word "healed" in this context does not refer to physical sickness. Instead, it points to a spiritual breach that needed divine correction. The people had approached a holy celebration without proper preparation, yet their hearts were sincere. God responded not with punishment, but with healing. This shows that healing in the Bible is not limited to the body—it includes spiritual restoration and the renewal of relationship with God.

The Hebrew word *rapha*, translated here as "healed," carries deep meaning. It refers not only to curing illness but also to restoring something to its proper and useful state. *Rapha* can describe physical recovery, but it also speaks of spiritual renewal, moral repair, and communal restoration. In this passage, *rapha* reflects God's grace in restoring worship, renewing hearts, and accepting imperfect people who seek Him sincerely.

This story reminds us that healing is often about more than health—it's about being made whole. When people turn to God with honest hearts, even if they fall short of ritual standards, He responds with mercy and restoration. Hezekiah's leadership, prayer, and trust in God's compassion opened the way for *rapha*—a healing that reached beyond rules and touched the soul. It is a powerful example of how divine healing brings people back into alignment with God's purpose and presence.

Chapter 19
Healed in the book of Psalms

1. Psalms 30:1-3

1 I will extol You, O Lord, for You have lifted me up, And have not let my foes rejoice over me.

2 O Lord my God, I cried out to You, And You healed me.

3 O Lord, You brought my soul up from the grave; You have kept me alive, that I should not go down to the pit.

Summary

This passage comes from a hymn of thanksgiving written by King David, where he expresses deep gratitude to God for delivering him from trouble. David praises the Lord for lifting him out of distress and not allowing his enemies to defeat him. In a moment of weakness and fear, David cried out to God, and God responded with mercy and healing. The Lord restored David's strength, protected his life, and saved him from the edge of death—described poetically as "the pit."

The hymn highlights David's personal experience of divine intervention, focusing on themes of restoration, protection, and God's faithful love. It stands as a powerful witness to the effectiveness of prayer and the kindness of God during times of suffering. David's story shows that healing in the biblical sense is not just about physical recovery—it is about being renewed in every way. It brings back life, purpose, and spiritual strength.

The word "healed" in this passage is based on the Hebrew term *rapha*, which usually means to cure or restore health. But *rapha* carries a deeper meaning. It refers to the process of making something whole again—repairing what is broken and returning it to its proper condition. This can apply to the body, the soul, relationships, or even circumstances. In David's case, *rapha* describes how God renewed his life, not just physically, but emotionally and spiritually.

The passage also quietly acknowledges the seriousness of illness and suffering. It suggests that without God's help, the natural outcome of such affliction could be death. Yet, through divine grace, that path can be changed. David's testimony shows that God's healing reaches far beyond physical pain— it touches the heart, lifts the spirit, and brings hope where there was despair.

This hymn reminds us that God's healing is complete and compassionate. It is not limited to curing disease but includes restoring joy, peace, and purpose. In every season of hardship, God remains present and willing to heal. Whether we face sickness, sorrow, or spiritual struggle, His power to *rapha*—to restore and renew—is always available.

David's words encourage us to trust in God's ability to heal all that is broken. His experience teaches that healing is not just relief—it is transformation. Through prayer, faith, and divine mercy, we too can experience the kind of renewal that brings life back into focus and restores us to the fullness of God's design.

2. Psalms 107:17-20

17 Fools, because of their transgression, And because of their iniquities, were afflicted.

18 Their soul abhorred all manner of food, And they drew near to the gates of death.

19 Then they cried out to the Lord in their trouble, And He saved them out of their distresses.

20 He sent His word and healed them, And delivered them from their destructions.

Summary

This passage offers a profound reflection on divine mercy and the restorative power of God's word. It portrays individuals who suffer as a direct consequence of their own transgressions and iniquities—described as "foolish" due to their disregard for righteousness. Their affliction leads them to a state of physical and spiritual decline, where even the basic desire for food fades, and they draw near to the gates of death.

In this desperate condition, they cry out to the Lord. In response, God intervenes—not with condemnation, but with compassion. He sends forth His word, a divine instrument of healing and deliverance, to rescue them from destruction. This act underscores the transformative power of repentance and the unwavering readiness of God to restore those who turn to Him with sincere hearts.

The passage highlights several key theological themes: the consequences of sin, the necessity of repentance, and the redemptive nature of divine intervention. It affirms that suffering, even when self-inflicted, is not beyond the reach of God's grace. His word does not merely alleviate symptoms; it restores wholeness and renews life.

The term "healed" in this context is derived from the Hebrew *rapha*, which traditionally means to heal or cure. However, its deeper significance encompasses rehabilitation, renovation, and the restoration of something to its original, functional state. In this passage, *rapha* conveys more than physical recovery—it speaks to the renewal of the soul, the mending of brokenness, and the reestablishment of purpose.

Ultimately, this text is a testament to God's enduring mercy and the power of His word to redeem, restore, and heal—even those who have wandered far from His ways.

Chapter 20
Healed in the book of Isaiah

1. Isaiah 6:8-10

8 Also I heard the voice of the Lord, saying: "Whom shall I send, And who will go for Us?" Then I said, "Here am I! Send me."

9 And He said, "Go, and tell this people: 'Keep on hearing, but do not understand;

Keep on seeing, but do not perceive.'

10 "Make the heart of this people dull, And their ears heavy, And shut their eyes;

Lest they see with their eyes, And hear with their ears, And understand with their heart, And return and be healed."

Summary

This passage describes a powerful moment in the life of the prophet Isaiah, occurring in the year King Uzziah died. Isaiah receives a vision of the Lord seated in glory within the temple, surrounded by heavenly beings called seraphim. Overwhelmed by the holiness of God, Isaiah becomes deeply aware of his own sinfulness and the brokenness of his people. He cries out, "Woe is me, for I am ruined! I am a man of unclean lips, and I live among a people of unclean lips; for my eyes have seen the King, the Lord of hosts."

In response to Isaiah's confession, one of the seraphim flies to him with a burning coal taken from the altar and touches his lips. This act symbolizes divine cleansing—God removing Isaiah's guilt and preparing him for service. With his sin forgiven, Isaiah responds to God's call with readiness and humility: "Here am I; send me."

God then gives Isaiah a difficult mission. He is to deliver a message that will reveal the spiritual blindness and stubbornness of the people of Israel. Isaiah is told to proclaim, "Keep on hearing, but do not understand; keep on seeing, but do not perceive." His words will not bring healing immediately, but instead will expose the depth of the people's resistance to God. They will hear the truth but refuse to respond, remaining distant from the healing that God desires to give.

This passage shows both Isaiah's willingness to serve and the seriousness of his prophetic task. It highlights the tension between God's desire to reveal Himself and the human tendency to reject that revelation. Isaiah's role is not only to speak but to participate in the unfolding of divine judgment, as the people's refusal to listen prevents them from being restored.

The word "healed" in this passage comes from the Hebrew *rapha*, which means more than just curing illness. It refers to restoring something to its proper and whole condition. In this context, *rapha* speaks of spiritual healing—a return to covenant faithfulness and renewed relationship with God. It is not just about physical health, but about the heart being made right.

Ultimately, this passage reminds us that healing begins with recognition of brokenness and a willingness to respond to God. Isaiah's cleansing and calling show that God is ready to restore, but healing—*rapha*—requires openness, repentance, and a heart willing to be changed.

2. Isaiah 53:4-5

4 Surely He has borne our griefs And carried our sorrows; Yet we esteemed Him stricken, Smitten by God, and afflicted.

5 But He was wounded for our transgressions, He was bruised for our iniquities;

The chastisement for our peace was upon Him, And by His stripes we are healed.

Summary

This passage, drawn from the prophetic writings of Isaiah, offers a profound and detailed vision of the coming Messiah—his appearance, mission, suffering, and ultimate redemptive work. Isaiah begins with a rhetorical question: "Who has believed our report?"—

underscoring the unexpected nature of the prophecy. Contrary to worldly expectations, the Messiah will not possess physical beauty or commanding presence. His appearance will be humble, his body frail, and his demeanor unremarkable. He will not attract followers through outward charm or stature.

Rather than being honored, he will be rejected and misunderstood. He will be deeply familiar with sorrow and suffering. People will look down on him, failing to see the divine purpose behind his pain. Yet Isaiah makes it clear that this suffering is not meaningless. It is purposeful and redemptive. The Messiah will carry the weight of human sin. He will be pierced for our wrongdoing and crushed for our failures. The punishment that brings peace to others will fall on him. And through his wounds, healing will be made possible.

This passage lays the foundation for the biblical idea of redemptive suffering. It points forward to Jesus Christ, who Christians believe fulfills this prophecy. His suffering and death are not just tragic events—they are the means by which healing and restoration are offered to the world. The healing described here is not only physical but also spiritual and relational.

The word "healed" in this passage comes from the Hebrew word *rapha*. While *rapha* can mean to cure illness, its meaning is much broader. It speaks of restoring something to its proper condition—repairing what is broken and making it whole again. In Isaiah's vision, *rapha* refers to the healing of humanity itself. It is not just about easing pain, but about restoring people to the life and relationship with God they were created for.

This kind of healing touches every part of life. It includes forgiveness, peace, and the renewal of purpose. The Messiah's suffering becomes the path through which broken lives are mended and people are brought back into right relationship with God.

Ultimately, this passage reminds us that true healing—*rapha*—comes through divine grace. It is not earned or deserved, but given through the sacrifice of the one who suffered in our place. Through him, healing is not only possible—it is promised.

Chapter 21
Healed in the book of Jeremiah

1. Jeremiah 6:11-14

11 Therefore I am full of the fury of the Lord. I am weary of holding it in. "I will pour it out on the children outside, And on the assembly of young men together; For even the husband shall be taken with the wife, The aged with him who is full of days.

12 And their houses shall be turned over to others, Fields and wives together; For I will stretch out My hand Against the inhabitants of the land," says the Lord.

13 "Because from the least of them even to the greatest of them, Everyone is given to covetousness; And from the prophet even to the priest, Everyone deals falsely.

14 They have also healed the hurt of My people slightly, Saying, 'Peace, peace!' When there is no peace.

Summary

This passage from the book of Jeremiah delivers a serious warning about God's coming judgment on Israel. The people had continued in sin, and their leaders—especially the prophets and priests—had led them astray. Instead of guiding the nation with truth and integrity, these leaders spread lies and offered false hope. They claimed everything was fine, saying "peace, peace," when there was no peace. Their words covered up the real problems, leaving the people's deep wounds untreated.

God's judgment, as described by Jeremiah, would affect everyone—young and old, rich and poor, leaders and common people. Homes, land, and families would be taken away and given to others. This shows how deeply the nation had fallen and how completely its society would be shaken. The warning is not just about punishment—it is about the consequences of ignoring truth and rejecting God's ways.

Jeremiah paints a picture of a society filled with corruption. From the lowest to the highest, people were acting dishonestly. Even those who were supposed to speak for God—the prophets and priests—were more concerned with their own gain than with the well-being of the people. They offered shallow solutions instead of real help. They did not deal with the root of the nation's problems. Instead, they gave easy answers that made things worse.

The word "healed" in this passage comes from the Hebrew word *rapha*. While *rapha* can mean physical healing, it also means much more. It speaks of restoring something to its proper, healthy condition—repairing what is broken and making it whole again. In this context, *rapha* is used to show what the leaders failed to do. They did not bring true healing. They did not help the people return to God or fix what was wrong in the nation.

Instead of leading the people toward real change, they covered up the truth. Their failure was not just a mistake—it was a betrayal of their responsibility to God and to the people. Jeremiah's message is clear: without true *rapha*—without real restoration—there can be no peace.

This passage calls for honest leadership and a return to God's ways. It reminds us that healing is not just about feeling better—it's about being made right. Only God can bring true *rapha*, and only when people are willing to face the truth and turn back to Him.

2. Jeremiah 8:10-11

10 Therefore I will give their wives to others, And their fields to those who will inherit them; Because from the least even to the greatest Everyone is given to covetousness; From the prophet even to the priest Everyone deals falsely.

11 For they have healed the hurt of the daughter of My people slightly, Saying, 'Peace, peace!' When there is no peace.

Summary

This passage from the book of Jeremiah repeats and strengthens a warning first given in chapter 6. The prophet speaks clearly about the ongoing sin of the people and the dishonesty of their leaders. Jeremiah announces that God's judgment is certain: families will lose their homes and fields, and everything they own will be handed over to others. This is the result of deep corruption and moral failure throughout the nation.

Greed has spread from the lowest to the highest levels of society. Even the prophets and priests—those who were supposed to guide the people in truth—have become part of the problem. Instead of speaking honestly, they tell the people everything is fine. They say "peace" when there is no peace. Their words offer comfort, but not healing. They cover up the real issues with quick fixes that do not last. Their concern is not for the people's well-being, but for their own gain.

These leaders fail to deal with the root causes of suffering. They do not call the people to repentance or lead them back to God. Instead, they offer shallow answers that leave the deeper wounds untouched. This shows a lack of integrity and spiritual wisdom. The hearts of the people have grown hard, and their leaders have lost sight of their true calling.

The passage is a strong message about the spiritual condition of Israel and the failure of its leadership. It warns of what happens when truth is replaced with lies and when God's wisdom is ignored. The word "healed" is used in an ironic way—it points to the false promises made by the leaders. They speak of healing, but they do not offer real restoration.

The Hebrew word *rapha*, translated as "healed," usually refers to physical healing. But its deeper meaning includes restoring something to its proper and healthy state. It speaks of renewal, repair, and making things whole again. In this passage, the absence of true *rapha* shows that the leaders are not helping the people. They are keeping them in a broken state.

Jeremiah's words are a call to turn back to God. Real healing—true *rapha*—comes only through repentance, truth, and divine grace. This passage reminds us that surface solutions are not enough. What is broken must be restored from the inside out. Only God can bring the kind of healing that renews hearts, communities, and nations.

3. Jeremiah 15:15-18

15 O Lord, You know; Remember me and visit me, And take vengeance for me on my persecutors. In Your enduring patience, do not take me away. Know that for Your sake I have suffered rebuke.

16 Your words were found, and I ate them, And Your word was to me the joy and rejoicing of my heart; For I am called by Your name, O Lord God of hosts.

17 I did not sit in the assembly of the mockers, Nor did I rejoice; I sat alone because of Your hand, For You have filled me with indignation.

18 Why is my pain perpetual And my wound incurable, Which refuses to be healed? Will You surely be to me like an unreliable stream, As waters that fail?

Summary

This passage presents a heartfelt and painful prayer from the prophet Jeremiah, who openly shares his suffering and frustration with God. He pleads for God to remember him, to come near, to protect him from death, and to bring justice against those who attack him. Jeremiah's cry is not based on self-pity but on his deep commitment to God's word and calling.

He reminds God that his pain comes from faithfully carrying out his prophetic mission. Jeremiah has fully embraced God's word—he says he "devoured" it, finding joy and delight in its truth. Because of this, he chose to separate himself from those who mocked and rejected God. He accepted loneliness and sorrow as part of his role, carrying the burden of God's message even when it brought him rejection and isolation.

Despite his devotion, Jeremiah ends his prayer with a cry of despair. He compares his pain to a wound that will not heal and expresses a deep sense of abandonment. He wonders why his suffering continues without relief. This moment shows Jeremiah's humanity—his vulnerability, his longing for healing, and his struggle to understand how his pain fits into God's plan.

The word "healed" in this passage comes from the Hebrew word *rapha*. While *rapha* often means physical healing, its deeper meaning includes restoration, renewal, and bringing something back to its proper and useful state. Jeremiah's use of *rapha* shows that his suffering is not just physical—it is emotional and spiritual. He feels broken inside, disconnected from God's presence and purpose.

This passage reveals the tension between being faithful to God and experiencing personal pain. Jeremiah shows that even the most committed servants of God can feel overwhelmed, discouraged, and in need of healing. His prayer is honest and raw, showing that it is okay to bring our deepest struggles to God.

Ultimately, Jeremiah's cry for healing is a longing for *rapha*—not just relief from pain, but full restoration. He wants to be renewed in spirit, reconnected to God, and restored to strength and purpose. This passage reminds us that divine healing reaches beyond the body. It touches the heart, the soul, and the calling of those who serve. Even in moments of despair, God's healing power is available to restore what feels lost and broken.

4. Jeremiah 17:14-15

14 Heal me, O Lord, and I shall be healed; Save me, and I shall be saved, For You are my praise.

15 Indeed they say to me, "Where is the word of the Lord? Let it come now!"

Summary

This passage shares a deeply personal prayer from the prophet Jeremiah, who cries out to God for healing and rescue. His words come from a place of pain, but also from deep trust. Jeremiah believes that only God can restore him—body, soul, and spirit. Even though people mock him and question whether God's judgment will ever come, Jeremiah does not lose faith. The doubters challenge his message and cast doubt on God's justice, but Jeremiah remains firm in his calling.

Instead of responding with anger, Jeremiah shows spiritual strength. He gives his pain, his reputation, and his future to God, trusting that the Lord will defend him in the right time. This moment shows both his vulnerability and his courage. Though rejected and misunderstood, Jeremiah continues to place his hope in God's faithfulness.

The passage highlights two important themes. First, it shows Jeremiah's steady trust in God, even when others laugh at him. Second, it reveals his frustration with people who refuse to take God's word seriously. Jeremiah's experience reminds us that true faith often means standing alone, holding on to God's promises even when others turn away.

The word "healed" in this passage comes from the Hebrew word *rapha*. While *rapha* can mean physical healing, its deeper meaning goes beyond that. It speaks of restoring something to its proper condition—repairing what is broken and making it whole again. In Jeremiah's prayer, healing is not just about feeling better. It's about being renewed in purpose, dignity, and strength.

Jeremiah's cry for healing shows that his suffering is more than physical. He feels the weight of rejection, loneliness, and spiritual struggle. He longs for God to restore him—not just to remove the pain, but to renew his sense of calling and connection with God. This kind of healing is full and deep. It reaches into the heart and brings life where there was despair.

This passage reminds us that God's healing—*rapha*—is not limited to curing illness. It includes restoring broken spirits, renewing lost purpose, and lifting those who feel crushed by life. Jeremiah's prayer is a powerful example of how faith holds on, even in the darkest moments, trusting that God can bring true healing and restoration.

5. Jeremiah 51:8-9

8 Babylon has suddenly fallen and been destroyed. Wail for her! Take balm for her pain; Perhaps she may be healed.

9 We would have healed Babylon, But she is not healed. Forsake her, and let us go everyone to his own country; For her judgment reaches to heaven and is lifted up to the skies.

Summary

This passage from the book of Jeremiah gives a serious and sorrowful message about the fall of Babylon. The prophet announces that Babylon's destruction will come quickly and cannot be stopped. He calls the people to mourn and offer incense—a symbolic act of comfort and healing. But this gesture is in vain. Jeremiah makes it clear that Babylon cannot be healed. Her condition is beyond repair, and the only option left is to leave her behind.

The images in this passage are strong and vivid. Babylon's judgment is said to reach the heavens, showing how complete and final God's decision is. This is not just the fall of a powerful city—it is a spiritual judgment. Babylon's long history of rebellion, pride, and corruption has pushed God's patience to its limit. The passage shows how serious divine justice is and how human efforts cannot fix what God has condemned.

At the heart of this prophecy is the word "healed," which comes from the Hebrew word *rapha*. While *rapha* often means to cure or restore health, it has a deeper meaning. It speaks of bringing something back to its proper and useful state—repairing, renewing, and making whole again. In this passage, the fact that Babylon cannot be *rapha*—cannot be healed—shows that her problems go far beyond politics or society. Her spiritual condition is broken, and no human plan can fix it.

Jeremiah's words remind us that some forms of brokenness are too deep for human solutions. Babylon's fall is not just a warning to one nation—it is a message to all who turn away from God. When corruption becomes a way of life and truth is rejected, healing becomes impossible. The failure to restore Babylon is not because God is unwilling, but because the time for mercy has passed and judgment must come.

This passage teaches a sobering truth: not all wounds can be healed, especially when they are caused by persistent defiance against God. It shows the limits of human power and the seriousness of divine justice. At the same time, it highlights the meaning of *rapha*—true healing is not just about fixing what is broken, but about restoring things to their rightful place under God's rule.

In the end, Jeremiah's prophecy is a call to listen, repent, and seek real healing before it's too late. Only God can bring true *rapha*, and only those who turn to Him will find restoration.

Chapter 22
Healed in the book of Ezekiel

1. Ezekiel 30:20-21 (KJV)

20 And it came to pass in the eleventh year, in the first month, in the seventh day of the month, that the word of the Lord came unto me, saying,

21 Son of man, I have broken the arm of Pharaoh king of Egypt; and, lo, it shall not be bound up to be healed, to put a roller to bind it, to make it strong to hold the sword.

Summary

This passage from the book of Ezekiel delivers a strong and symbolic message of judgment against Pharaoh, the king of Egypt. God declares that He has broken Pharaoh's arm—a powerful image that represents the collapse of Egypt's military strength and political control. What makes this judgment even more serious is that the arm will not be bandaged or healed. It will not be restored to hold a sword again. This shows that Egypt's fall will be permanent, and recovery will not be possible.

The broken arm is more than just a physical injury. It stands for Egypt's complete loss of power and influence. Once a mighty nation, Egypt will become weak and unable to protect itself or lead others. The fact that God refuses to heal or strengthen Pharaoh's arm highlights the totality of His judgment. There will be no second chance, no return to greatness, and no escape from the consequences.

This passage reminds us of God's ultimate authority over all nations and rulers. No human power can stand against His will. Egypt's downfall is not due to bad luck or poor leadership—it is the result of God's decision. This serves as a warning to anyone who puts their trust in human strength instead of relying on God. When a nation turns away from Him, even its strongest leaders cannot prevent its collapse.

The word "healed" in this passage comes from the Hebrew word *rephu'ah*, which means remedy, medicine, or cure. It is related to the verb *rapha*, meaning "to heal." But *rephu'ah* goes beyond just treating sickness. It speaks of restoring something to its proper, working condition—whether that's a body, a nation, or a relationship. It includes physical, emotional, and spiritual renewal.

In Ezekiel's prophecy, the absence of *rephu'ah* shows that Egypt's condition is beyond repair. God has chosen not to restore what He has broken. This is not just about losing battles—it is about losing the chance for healing and renewal. Egypt's judgment is final, and no human effort can reverse it.

This passage is a powerful reminder that true healing—*rephu'ah*—comes only from God. When He chooses to restore, it brings life and strength. But when He withholds healing, even the strongest nations fall. It calls us to trust in God's authority and seek His restoration before it's too late.

2. Ezekiel 34:1-4

1 And the word of the Lord came to me, saying,

2 "Son of man, prophesy against the shepherds of Israel, prophesy and say to them, 'Thus says the Lord God to the shepherds: "Woe to the shepherds of Israel who feed themselves! Should not the shepherds feed the flocks?

3 You eat the fat and clothe yourselves with the wool; you slaughter the fatlings, but you do not feed the flock.

4 The weak you have not strengthened, nor have you healed those who were sick, nor bound up the broken, nor brought back what was driven away, nor sought what was lost; but with force and cruelty you have ruled them.

Summary

This passage from the book of Ezekiel delivers a strong message from God against the leaders of Israel, who are described as shepherds. Instead of caring for the people, these leaders acted selfishly. They enjoyed the good things of the land but ignored those who were weak, sick, or injured. They did not help those who had wandered away or try to find those who were lost. In doing so, they failed in their responsibility to guide and protect the people.

God's accusation is clear: these leaders have turned away from their calling. They were supposed to feed, heal, and care for the people, but instead they caused harm. Their actions led to suffering and scattered the people, leaving them vulnerable and without direction. This passage reveals the deep moral and spiritual failure of Israel's leadership and prepares the way for God to step in.

In response to this failure, God announces that He Himself will become the shepherd of His people. He will gather those who have been scattered, heal those who are wounded, and bring justice to those who have been mistreated. This promise brings hope. It shows that God will not leave His people in the hands of corrupt leaders. Instead, He will take personal responsibility for their care and restoration.

The word "healed" in this passage comes from the Hebrew word *rapha*. While *rapha* often means to cure sickness, it also has a deeper meaning. It refers to restoring something to its proper and healthy condition. It includes physical healing, but also emotional, spiritual, and social renewal. In Ezekiel's message, healing is not just about fixing injuries—it is about making the people whole again after being hurt and abandoned.

God's promise to heal shows His desire to bring full restoration. He will not only mend broken bodies but also repair broken hearts, rebuild trust, and restore dignity. The people have been betrayed by their leaders, but God will bring them back to safety and purpose. His healing—*rapha*—is complete and life-giving.

This passage reminds us that true leadership cares for others, and that God's healing reaches every part of life. When human leaders fail, God remains faithful. He sees the pain, hears the cries, and acts with compassion. Through *rapha*, He restores what is broken and brings His people back to wholeness.

3. Ezekiel 47:7-12

7 When I returned, there, along the bank of the river, were very many trees on one side and the other.

8 Then he said to me: "This water flows toward the eastern region, goes down into the valley, and enters the sea. When it reaches the sea, its waters are healed.

9 And it shall be that every living thing that moves, wherever the rivers go, will live. There will be a very great multitude of fish, because these waters go there; for they will be healed, and everything will live wherever the river goes.

10 It shall be that fishermen will stand by it from En Gedi to En Eglaim; they will be places for spreading their nets. Their fish will be of the same kinds as the fish of the Great Sea, exceedingly many.

11 But its swamps and marshes will not be healed; they will be given over to salt.

12 Along the bank of the river, on this side and that, will grow all kinds of trees used for food; their leaves will not wither, and their fruit will not fail. They will bear fruit every month, because their water flows from the sanctuary. Their fruit will be for food, and their leaves for medicine."

Summary

This passage from the book of Ezekiel describes a powerful vision of healing and restoration that flows directly from God's presence. The prophet is led back to the entrance of the temple, where he sees water coming out from beneath the threshold, heading east. As he walks through the water at measured intervals, it gradually becomes deeper—first reaching his ankles, then his knees, then his waist—until it grows into a mighty river too deep to cross.

Since the river cannot be crossed, Ezekiel is brought back to its banks. There, he sees trees growing on both sides, full of life. His guide explains that the water will flow through the eastern region, into the valley, and finally into the sea. When it reaches the sea, something amazing happens—the salty waters are healed. Wherever this river flows, it brings life. Plants grow, animals thrive, and communities are renewed. Fishermen will gather many kinds of fish, and the trees along the river will bear fruit every month. Their leaves will never dry up, and their fruit will never fail.

This vision is a picture of the healing power that comes from God. The water flowing from the temple stands for God's grace—pure, life-giving, and full of renewal. Even though it starts as a small stream, it grows into a powerful river that transforms everything it touches. It shows how God's presence brings healing not just to individuals, but to the land, the sea, and all living things.

For those who follow God, this vision offers a message of hope. Just as the river brings life wherever it flows, people who stay close to God and are nourished by His word can bring healing and renewal to others. It reminds us that great change often begins in small ways, but when connected to God, it grows and bears lasting fruit.

The word "healed" in this passage comes from the Hebrew word *rapha*. While *rapha* can mean physical healing, it also refers to restoring something to its proper and useful state. It includes renewal, repair, and making things whole again. In Ezekiel's vision, *rapha* is not just about curing sickness—it's about restoring life, purpose, and balance to everything that has been broken.

This passage encourages us to trust in the healing flow of God's grace. When we stay connected to Him, we become part of His work to restore the world.

Chapter 23
Healed in the book of Hosea

1. Hosea 7:1-3

1 "When I would have healed Israel, Then the iniquity of Ephraim was uncovered, And the wickedness of Samaria. For they have committed fraud; A thief comes in; A band of robbers takes spoil outside.

2 They do not consider in their hearts That I remember all their wickedness; Now their own deeds have surrounded them; They are before My face.

3 They make a king glad with their wickedness, And princes with their lies.

Summary

This passage gives a serious look at the spiritual condition of Israel, showing how deeply the people have turned away from God. Corruption and moral failure are everywhere. God clearly wants to heal and restore His people, but their ongoing sin blocks the way. Acts of theft, dishonesty, and abuse are committed without any fear of God or concern for His judgment. The people act as if God does not see or care about their wrongdoing.

These sins are not just personal—they are widespread and accepted by those in power. Leaders like kings and princes enjoy these injustices and help them grow. The nation's rebellion is not hidden; it is celebrated. The weight of Israel's sin has become so great that it forms a barrier between them and the healing God wants to give. Restoration is held back—not because God refuses to help, but because the people will not turn from their sin or open their eyes to the truth.

This passage shows how important repentance is for restoration. Healing from God is not just about fixing problems or easing pain. It is about restoring relationships, renewing purpose, and bringing people back to the life God intended. The Hebrew word *rapha*, often translated as "healed," means more than curing sickness. It speaks of repairing, rebuilding, and returning something to its proper and useful state.

In this context, *rapha* is about restoring Israel's covenant with God. It is not just physical healing—it is spiritual renewal. God wants to bring His people back to Himself, but they must be willing to change. Healing is available, but it is not automatic. It requires humility, honesty, and a desire to confront sin.

Israel's refusal to repent serves as a warning. When people choose corruption and ignore God's judgment, even His desire to heal cannot undo the damage of hardened hearts. Restoration does not begin with

God alone—it begins when people respond to His truth.

This passage reminds us that God's grace is always ready, but we must be willing to receive it. Healing—*rapha*—comes when we turn from sin and open our hearts to God. Only then can we be restored to the life and purpose He has planned.

2. Hosea 11:1-3

1 "When Israel was a child, I loved him, And out of Egypt I called My son.

2 As they called them, So they went from them; They sacrificed to the Baals, And burned incense to carved images.

3 "I taught Ephraim to walk, Taking them by their arms; But they did not know that I healed them.

Summary

This passage paints a moving picture of God's deep sorrow over Israel's repeated rejection of His love. God is shown as a caring and faithful Father who remembers calling His people out of Egypt and guiding them with tenderness. He provided for them, protected them, and brought healing to their lives. His relationship with Israel was built on closeness and compassion. Yet, despite all this, the people turned away. They chose idols and rebellion instead of staying faithful to the covenant. They forgot the One who had healed and sustained them.

Even in the face of this betrayal, God does not respond with anger or abandonment. Instead, He continues to reach out with love and mercy. He offers kindness and grace, longing to restore the broken relationship. His desire to heal remains strong, showing the depth of His compassion. God's love is not based on how perfect His people are—it flows from who He is: patient, merciful, and committed to restoration.

The Hebrew word for "healed" in this passage is *rapha*. While *rapha* often means to cure illness, it carries a richer meaning. It speaks of restoring something to its proper and useful state—repairing what is broken, renewing what has been damaged, and bringing things back to how they were meant to be. In this context, God's healing is not just physical. It is relational and spiritual. He wants to bring Israel back to its true identity as His beloved people.

This vision of healing shows that God's grace is always available, even when His people have strayed far from Him. He does not give up. Instead, He keeps calling them back, offering to heal what has been wounded and to renew what has been lost. His love goes beyond offense. It seeks reconciliation, not revenge.

This passage is a powerful reminder of God's faithfulness. It tells us that no matter how far we fall, God's desire is to restore us. His healing—*rapha*—is complete. It touches every part of life: body, heart, and soul. It brings us back into relationship with Him and renews our purpose.

Even today, this message offers hope. God's love is steady, and His healing is real. When we turn to Him, He is ready to restore what is broken and lead us into wholeness once again.

PART 3

HEALER IN THE OLD TESTAMENT

Chapter 24
Healer in the book of Isaiah

1. Isaiah 3:6-8

6 When a man shall take hold of his brother of the house of his father, saying, Thou hast clothing, be thou our ruler, and let this ruin be under thy hand:

7 In that day shall he swear, saying, I will not be an healer; for in my house is neither bread nor clothing: make me not a ruler of the people.

8 For Jerusalem is ruined, and Judah is fallen: because their tongue and their doings are against the Lord, to provoke the eyes of his glory.

Summary

This passage from the book of Isaiah gives a serious warning about the coming judgment on Jerusalem and the kingdom of Judah. Isaiah describes a time of deep trouble, where society is falling apart and spiritual values have been lost. People are desperate for leadership, but no one is willing or able to take charge. In one scene, a man grabs his brother and says, "You have clothing—be our leader and take control of this mess." The request isn't based on wisdom or skill. It's based on appearance alone, showing how hopeless things have become. People are looking for anyone who seems to have something, even if it's just clothes.

The word "healer" in this passage comes from the Hebrew word *chabash*. It means to bind, wrap, or bandage a wound. It can also mean to comfort, to restore, or even to lead and govern. So when someone says, "I am not a healer," they're saying, "I can't fix this. I can't lead. I can't restore what's broken."

The brother's response is powerful: "Don't make me your leader. I'm not a healer, and I don't even have bread or clothing." He's admitting that he has nothing to offer—not even the basics. He knows he can't help, and he refuses the role. This isn't just about one man. It shows a bigger truth: when a nation turns away from God, no human leader can fix the damage. The problem is spiritual, and human solutions aren't enough.

Isaiah makes it clear that the downfall of Jerusalem and Judah is because they rejected God. Their actions and words have gone against God's commands and have insulted His glory. This rebellion isn't quiet or hidden—it's bold and open. And the result is destruction. Isaiah's message is strong: when people ignore God's authority and holiness, they bring disaster on themselves.

This passage teaches two important lessons:

- **The Results of Sin**: The collapse of Judah and Jerusalem is a direct result of their rebellion. Their behavior has broken their relationship with God, and now they face judgment. Isaiah warns that sin doesn't just hurt individuals—it can tear apart entire communities.

- **Human Efforts Fall Short**: In the middle of the chaos, even those who seem capable refuse to lead. The brother's words—"I am not a healer"—show that fixing spiritual problems takes more than human strength. Bread and clothing, symbols of care and dignity, are missing. Real healing must come from God.

Isaiah's words challenge us to think about what true leadership looks like and where real healing comes from. In times of crisis, when human plans fail, this passage reminds us that restoration begins with turning back to God—with humility, repentance, and trust in His power to *chabash*—to bind up what has been broken and make it whole again.

PART 4

HEALS IN THE OLD TESTAMENT

Chapter 25
Heals in the book of Exodus

1. Exodus 15:24-27

24 And the people complained against Moses, saying, "What shall we drink?"

25 So he cried out to the Lord, and the Lord showed him a tree. When he cast it into the waters, the waters were made sweet. There He made a statute and an ordinance for them, and there He tested them,

26 and said, "If you diligently heed the voice of the Lord your God and do what is right in His sight, give ear to His commandments and keep all His statutes, I will put none of the diseases on you which I have brought on the Egyptians. For I am the Lord who heals you."

27 Then they came to Elim, where there were twelve wells of water and seventy palm trees; so they camped there by the waters.

Summary

After three days of arduous travel through the desert, the Israelites—newly freed from Egyptian bondage—

found themselves in desperate need of water. Their journey led them to a place called Marah, where they finally discovered water. However, their relief was short-lived. The waters of Marah were bitter and undrinkable, a cruel twist in their already difficult journey. The name "Marah," meaning "bitterness," was aptly given to reflect both the physical condition of the water and the emotional state of the people.

Faced with this disappointment, the people quickly turned against Moses, voicing their frustration and fear. Their question—"What shall we drink?"—was not merely logistical; it revealed a deeper spiritual unrest. Despite witnessing God's miraculous deliverance from Egypt, they faltered in faith at the first sign of adversity. Their murmuring against Moses was, in essence, a rejection of God's provision and a failure to trust His guidance.

In contrast to the people's reaction, Moses responded with humility and dependence. He turned to the Lord for direction, seeking divine wisdom rather than relying on human solutions. God answered by showing Moses a specific tree, instructing him to throw it into the bitter waters. Moses obeyed without hesitation, and the water was miraculously transformed—sweetened and made fit for consumption. This act was not only a physical remedy but a spiritual signpost, revealing God's power to heal and restore.

It was at Marah that God used the moment to test His people and establish a conditional covenant. He declared, "If you diligently listen to the voice of the

Lord your God and do what is right in His eyes, and pay attention to His commandments and keep all His statutes, I will not bring upon you any of the diseases I brought upon the Egyptians. For I am the Lord who heals you." This covenant was both a promise and a challenge: obedience would lead to divine protection and healing, while disobedience would invite consequences.

The Hebrew word used for "heals" in this passage is *raphah*, a term rich with layered meaning. While commonly translated as "to heal," *raphah* also conveys the ideas of relaxing, letting go, ceasing to struggle, and withdrawing. It suggests a posture of surrender—an invitation to release control and allow God to act. In some contexts, *raphah* is associated with weakness or helplessness, emphasizing the need for divine intervention. In this passage, healing is not merely physical; it is holistic, encompassing emotional, spiritual, and relational restoration.

To fully grasp the significance of *raphah*, one must consider the image of a person so identified with their affliction that they cannot release it. Healing, then, becomes an act of divine disruption—God forcibly removing the illness, breaking the bond of suffering, and restoring wholeness. It is a reminder that true healing often requires surrender, a relinquishing of self-reliance in favor of divine grace.

Following their experience at Marah, the Israelites journeyed to Elim, a place of abundance and refreshment. There they found twelve springs of water and seventy palm trees—a stark contrast to the bitterness of Marah. Elim represented God's intended destination for His people, a place of provision and peace. The temporary solution at Marah was never the final plan; it was a stepping stone, a test, and a lesson in trust.

This passage underscores several key truths:

- **The Rebellion of the People**: Despite witnessing God's mighty acts, the Israelites quickly forgot His faithfulness. Their complaints at Marah reveal how easily fear can overshadow faith when circumstances become difficult.

- **God's Faithfulness in the Face of Doubt**: Even as the people rebelled, God remained true to His character. He provided a solution to their immediate need and continued to guide them toward greater blessings.

- **God's Plans Surpass Human Imagination**: The contrast between Marah and Elim illustrates that God's ultimate provision far exceeds what we expect. What may seem like a bitter trial is often a prelude to divine abundance.

In essence, Marah was not just a geographical location—it was a spiritual crossroads. It revealed the fragility of human faith, the necessity of obedience, and the depth of God's healing power. Through *raphah*, we are reminded that healing begins when we let go, trust fully, and allow God to be our restorer.

Chapter 26
Heals in the book of Psalms

1. Psalms 103:1-5

1 Bless the Lord, O my soul; And all that is within me, bless His holy name!

2 Bless the Lord, O my soul, And forget not all His benefits:

3 Who forgives all your iniquities, Who heals all your diseases,

4 Who redeems your life from destruction, Who crowns you with lovingkindness and tender mercies,

5 Who satisfies your mouth with good things, So that your youth is renewed like the eagle's.

Summary

This passage, drawn from Psalm 103, offers a deeply personal and reflective moment in which King David engages in a dialogue with his own soul. He begins by commanding himself—his innermost being—to bless the Lord and to remember all His benefits. This is not a casual encouragement but a deliberate act of spiritual discipline, urging the soul to remain mindful of God's goodness and to respond with heartfelt praise.

David then proceeds to recount the manifold blessings he has received from God, presenting a rich tapestry of divine acts that touch every dimension of human life. He begins with the forgiveness of sins, acknowledging that God's mercy cleanses and restores the soul. This foundational act of grace sets the tone for the rest of the psalm, as David moves from spiritual renewal to physical restoration.

He declares that God heals all his diseases—a statement that encompasses both physical ailments and deeper emotional or spiritual afflictions. The Hebrew word used here for "heals" is *raphah*, which conveys the idea of repairing, restoring, and making whole. It suggests not only the removal of sickness but the reestablishment of health and vitality. In this context, healing is not limited to the body; it extends to every area of brokenness within the human experience.

David continues by celebrating God's redemptive power, noting that the Lord rescues his life from destruction. This speaks to divine intervention in moments of danger, despair, or spiritual peril. God does not merely preserve life—He redeems it, giving it purpose and direction. Following this, David describes being crowned with lovingkindness and tender mercies, a poetic image that reflects honor, favor, and the intimate compassion of God.

He also speaks of being satisfied with good things, a reference to divine provision and abundance. This satisfaction leads to renewal, as David likens his rejuvenation to that of the eagle—a creature known for its strength, longevity, and ability to soar. The metaphor suggests that God's blessings not only sustain but invigorate, enabling the believer to rise above adversity with renewed energy and perspective.

What emerges from this passage is a portrait of God's comprehensive care. His blessings are not confined to material prosperity; they encompass spiritual cleansing, emotional healing, physical restoration, and relational grace. David's testimony affirms that God is not only a healer but also a restorer, redeemer, and sustainer. These gifts are not earned through human merit but are freely given through divine grace.

In Psalm 103, David models a posture of gratitude and reverence. By instructing his soul to bless the Lord and remember His benefits, he invites all believers to cultivate a spirit of worship rooted in reflection. This passage reminds us that true praise flows from a heart that recognizes the depth and breadth of God's goodness—a goodness that touches every part of our lives and draws us into deeper communion with Him.

2. Psalms 147:1-3

1 Praise the Lord! For it is good to sing praises to our God; For it is pleasant, and praise is beautiful.

2 The Lord builds up Jerusalem; He gathers together the outcasts of Israel.

3 He heals the brokenhearted And binds up their wounds.

Summary

Psalm 147 opens with a heartfelt invitation from David to celebrate and praise the Lord. He reminds us that it is both good and fitting to offer praise to God—a practice that brings joy to the soul and honors the One who is the source of all goodness. This psalm is not merely a poetic reflection; it is a call to recognize the character and actions of God and to respond with sincere worship.

David highlights several divine attributes and interventions that warrant our praise. He declares that it is the Lord who rebuilds Jerusalem, a symbol of restoration and hope. In gathering the exiles of Israel, God demonstrates His commitment to reconciliation and unity, bringing His people back from dispersion and despair. These acts are not only historical but deeply spiritual, reflecting God's ongoing work of restoration in the lives of His people.

One of the most tender and powerful images in this passage is that of God healing the brokenhearted and binding up their wounds. This portrayal of divine compassion speaks to the depth of God's care for the vulnerable and afflicted. The Hebrew word used for "heals" is *raphah*, which encompasses a broad spectrum of meaning: to heal, to repair, to restore. It is a word that implies wholeness, not just the absence of pain. In this context, *raphah* refers to the complete healing God offers—physical, emotional, moral, and spiritual.

God's healing is not limited to one dimension of life. It touches every area of dysfunction and brokenness: our bodies, our relationships, our finances, and even our sense of purpose. Where there is fragmentation, God brings restoration. Where there is sorrow, He offers comfort. Where there is weakness, He imparts strength. This holistic healing reflects the fullness of God's grace and His desire for our flourishing.

The psalm also underscores the appropriate response to such divine mercy: praise. Worship is not merely a ritual or obligation—it is the natural outpouring of a grateful heart. When we reflect on all that God has done—redeeming us, restoring us, healing us—it becomes clear that praise is the most fitting and complete response. It aligns our hearts with God's goodness and reminds us of His faithfulness.

In essence, Psalm 147 is a celebration of God's restorative power and compassionate nature. It calls us to remember that every good thing in our lives—every moment of healing, every act of redemption—is a gift from God. And in light of that truth, we are invited to respond with joy, gratitude, and worship. David's words remind us that praise is not only good—it is essential, for it connects us to the heart of the One who heals, restores, and sustains us.

Chapter 27
Heals in the book of Isaiah

1. Isaiah 30:23-26

23 Then He will give the rain for your seed With which you sow the ground, And bread of the increase of the earth; It will be fat and plentiful. In that day your cattle will feed In large pastures.

24 Likewise the oxen and the young donkeys that work the ground Will eat cured fodder, Which has been winnowed with the shovel and fan.

25 There will be on every high mountain And on every high hill Rivers and streams of waters, In the day of the great slaughter, When the towers fall.

26 Moreover the light of the moon will be as the light of the sun, And the light of the sun will be sevenfold, As the light of seven days, In the day that the Lord binds up the bruise of His people And heals the stroke of their wound.

Summary

Following a period of divine condemnation for Israel's rebellion, the Lord instructs the prophet

Isaiah to record a prophetic declaration of grace and restoration. Despite the people's disobedience, God reveals His intention to renew and bless them abundantly. This passage unfolds as a vision of comprehensive restoration—one that touches every facet of creation and human life.

God's promises are both agricultural and spiritual in nature. He pledges to send rain upon the seeds sown by the people, ensuring that the land yields an abundant harvest. This divine provision reflects not only material prosperity but also a return to fruitfulness after a season of drought and judgment. The blessing extends to livestock as well, with a promise of flourishing herds. Even the working animals—oxen and donkeys—are included in this vision of abundance, receiving the finest hay and grain as nourishment for their labor.

The restoration continues with a vivid image of rivers and streams flowing freely from every mountain and hill. These waters will not run dry, symbolizing both physical sustenance and spiritual renewal. Water, often a biblical metaphor for life and cleansing, becomes a sign of God's enduring presence and care. The land, once parched and desolate, will be revitalized under divine provision.

One of the most striking elements of this prophecy is the transformation of light itself. God promises to increase the intensity and duration of daylight, such that the light of the moon will resemble that of the sun, and a single day will shine with the brightness of seven. This supernatural amplification of light suggests a return to Edenic conditions—a resetting of creation in favor of Israel. It evokes themes of divine glory, healing, and the removal of darkness, both literal and metaphorical.

Finally, God declares that He will bind up the wounds of His people and heal their afflictions. This promise of healing is deeply personal and communal. The Hebrew word often used in this context is *raphah*, which conveys the idea of repairing, restoring, and making whole. It encompasses physical healing, emotional restoration, and moral renewal. God's healing is not partial—it is holistic, addressing every area of brokenness within the nation.

This passage reveals a profound truth: divine restoration is not limited to spiritual reconciliation but extends to the environment, economy, and physical well-being of God's people. It is a vision of total renewal, where creation itself responds to the grace of God. The soil, the animals, the waters, and even the light are transformed to reflect divine favor.

In essence, Isaiah's prophecy presents a portrait of God's mercy triumphing over judgment. It affirms that, even after rebellion, restoration is possible through divine grace. God not only forgives—He renews, heals, and reorders creation to bless His people. This holistic vision invites us to trust in the fullness of God's redemptive power.

PART 5

HEALING IN THE OLD TESTAMENT

Chapter 28
Healing in the book of Jeremiah

1. Jeremiah 14:19-20

19 Have You utterly rejected Judah? Has Your soul loathed Zion? Why have You stricken us so that there is no healing for us? We looked for peace, but there was no good; And for the time of healing, and there was trouble.

20 We acknowledge, O Lord, our wickedness And the iniquity of our fathers, For we have sinned against You.

Summary

This passage presents a profoundly emotional moment in the ministry of the prophet Jeremiah, as he intercedes for the people of Judah amid the weight of divine judgment. Confronted with the severity of God's response to the nation's persistent rebellion, Jeremiah pleads with heartfelt urgency, asking whether Judah has been utterly rejected and whether Zion—once a symbol of divine favor—has become an object of contempt. His questions reflect both anguish and reverence, revealing a prophet who seeks not only answers but restoration.

Jeremiah's lament is far more than rhetorical; it is a sincere cry for mercy. He questions the intensity of God's judgment, wondering why the people have been struck so severely, seemingly without the opportunity to recover. The prophet observes that Judah had hoped for peace and healing, yet received only calamity and sorrow. Their expectations were crushed, and their wounds remained unhealed. This stark contrast between hope and reality underscores the depth of spiritual desolation and the consequences of covenantal unfaithfulness.

In this moment of intercession, Jeremiah does more than speak on behalf of the people—he identifies with their suffering and guilt. He acknowledges not only the sins of the present generation but also the iniquities of their ancestors. This recognition of generational transgression reveals a profound understanding of collective responsibility before God. His prayer is marked by humility and repentance, as he confesses the nation's failure to uphold the covenant and earnestly seeks divine forgiveness.

Several key theological themes emerge from this passage:

- **Divine Judgment in Response to Persistent Sin**: God's wrath is portrayed not as impulsive, but as a measured and just response to Judah's continued disobedience. The people's rejection of divine instruction and moral decline have led to grave consequences, demonstrating the seriousness of covenant violation.

- **Prophetic Intercession and Identification**: Jeremiah's role as prophet transcends proclamation. He becomes a mediator, standing between God and the people with empathy, sorrow, and solidarity. His intercession reflects the heart of a shepherd who shares in the suffering of those he represents.

- **Repentance and Recognition of Iniquity**: Restoration begins with honest confession. Jeremiah's acknowledgment of both personal and ancestral sin illustrates the depth of true repentance. It is not limited to individual guilt but encompasses the broader impact of generational failure.

- **The Social and Generational Consequences of Sin**: Sin's effects are never isolated. They ripple through families, communities, and future generations. Jeremiah's prayer echoes the urgency of collective repentance, as seen in the example of Nineveh (Jonah 3:5–10), where communal humility led to divine mercy.

The Hebrew word *marpe*, translated as "healing," conveys the idea of remedy, treatment, and restoration—both physical and spiritual. In this context, it evokes the longing for a season of renewal and divine intervention.

Ultimately, Jeremiah's intercession stands as a testament to the power of prayer and the hope of reconciliation. Even in the midst of judgment, he dares to seek healing, trusting in the compassion of a God who listens to the cries of a repentant people.

2. Jeremiah 30:12-15

12 "For thus says the Lord: 'Your affliction is incurable, Your wound is severe.

13 There is no one to plead your cause, That you may be bound up; You have no healing medicines.

14 All your lovers have forgotten you; They do not seek you; For I have wounded you with the wound of an enemy, With the chastisement of a cruel one, For the multitude of your iniquities, Because your sins have increased.

15 Why do you cry about your affliction? Your sorrow is incurable. Because of the multitude of your iniquities, Because your sins have increased, I have done these things to you.

Summary

In this solemn passage from the book of Jeremiah, the prophet delivers a piercing message of divine judgment upon Israel and the kingdom of Judah. Speaking on behalf of the Lord, Jeremiah unveils the depth of the nation's spiritual and moral collapse. The imagery is stark and uncompromising: the people's condition is described as incurable, their wounds too deep to be healed. This is not a temporary affliction, but a profound and entrenched crisis brought about by persistent rebellion against God.

The Lord declares that the people are forsaken—without an advocate to plead their cause and without a remedy to restore their health. Their allies, metaphorically referred to as lovers, have abandoned them, refusing to intervene or offer support. This abandonment intensifies the severity of their plight, highlighting the isolation and vulnerability that result from divine judgment. The Lord, once their protector, now stands as their adversary, having inflicted punishment for the multitude of their transgressions.

One of the most striking elements of this passage is God's rhetorical question: "Why do you weep over your wound?" This is not a dismissal of their suffering, but a sobering reminder that their grief is the direct consequence of their iniquity. Their sorrow is not unjust; it is the fruit of their rebellion. God affirms that He is the source of their suffering—not out of cruelty, but as a righteous response to their defiance of His covenant.

This passage reveals two profound theological truths:

- **The Consequences of Sin:** The judgment pronounced on Judah is not arbitrary or impulsive. It is the result of sustained disobedience and moral decay. Sin, when left unchecked, provokes divine wrath and leads to inevitable crisis. The incurable nature of the people's condition reflects the depth of their estrangement from God. Their wounds are not superficial—they are spiritual, systemic, and rooted in generations of rebellion.

- **Human Powerlessness in the Face of Divine Judgment:** Once divine judgment is enacted, no human effort can reverse it. The absence of defenders and remedies underscores the futility of relying on secular or superficial solutions to address spiritual problems. Restoration is possible, but only through sincere repentance and submission to God's will.

Jeremiah's message is not merely a condemnation—it is a call to reflection and repentance. It invites the reader to confront the gravity of sin and the urgent need for divine mercy. The incurable wound is not a final verdict, but a revelation of the depth of the problem. Healing remains possible, but only through the grace of God, who wounds in justice and heals in mercy.

The Hebrew word Te'alah, translated here as "healing," primarily refers to a watercourse or channel. In its figurative usage, it denotes a dressing or bandage applied to a wound—something that channels the healing process. In this context, the figurative meaning prevails, symbolizing the hope that even deep wounds can be tended and restored through divine intervention.

Chapter 29
Healing in the book of Nahum

1. Nahum 3:18-19

18 Your shepherds slumber, O king of Assyria; Your nobles rest in the dust. Your people are scattered on the mountains, And no one gathers them.

19 Your injury has no healing, Your wound is severe. All who hear news of you

Will clap their hands over you, For upon whom has not your wickedness passed continually?

Summary

In this compelling passage from the Book of Nahum, the prophet delivers a solemn and unambiguous pronouncement of divine judgment against Nineveh, the formidable capital of the Assyrian Empire. Once renowned for its military prowess, political dominance, and ruthless oppression, Nineveh now stands on the brink of irreversible collapse. Through Nahum, God declares that the time of reckoning has arrived, and the city's downfall will be complete and irrevocable.

The prophecy begins with a stark revelation: the city's shepherds and nobles—key figures in its leadership and societal stability—are dead. The shepherds, symbolic of laborers and agricultural providers, are no longer present to sustain the population. The nobles, representing the intellectual and administrative elite, have perished, leaving behind a vacuum of wisdom, governance, and strategic direction. Without these foundational pillars, the people are left to wander aimlessly in the mountains, disoriented and leaderless. The absence of leadership plunges Nineveh into chaos, stripping it of order, protection, and identity.

The imagery intensifies as God describes Nineveh's wound as incurable. This affliction is not superficial or temporary—it is deep, fatal, and beyond remedy. No physician, alliance, or human intervention can reverse the damage. The wound, both literal and symbolic, reflects the city's entrenched moral and spiritual decay. For generations, Nineveh's pride and arrogance have masked its vulnerability. Now, in its moment of collapse, it finds no comfort, no healing, and no escape. Its strength has become its downfall, and its refusal to repent has sealed its fate.

What makes this prophecy particularly striking is the reaction of the surrounding nations. Rather than mourning Nineveh's destruction, they rejoice. The text reveals that all who hear of its desolation celebrate, for they have long suffered under its cruelty. The fall of Nineveh is not merely a geopolitical event—it is a moment of vindication for the oppressed. The city, once a source of terror, becomes a public demonstration of divine justice. God's judgment affirms that He does not ignore wickedness or the cries of those crushed by injustice.

This passage brings to light several profound theological themes:

- **The Collapse of Human Systems**: The destruction of Nineveh's leaders signifies the dismantling of its societal infrastructure. Without its intellectual, economic, and political foundations, the city is exposed and vulnerable, unable to sustain itself.

- **The Humbling of Human Arrogance**: The incurable wound is a direct blow to Nineveh's pride. Its inability to heal itself underscores the futility of human strength when confronted with divine judgment.

- **The Certainty of Divine Justice**: God's judgment is not impulsive or arbitrary. It is a measured response to persistent wickedness and exploitation. The powerful are held accountable, and justice is ultimately served.

- **God's Advocacy for the Oppressed**: The rejoicing of the nations testifies to God's faithfulness. He hears the cries of the afflicted and acts on their behalf. The fall of Nineveh becomes a beacon of hope for all who suffer injustice, affirming that God sees, remembers, and will bring justice in His time.

The Hebrew word *kēhâh*, translated here as "healing," carries layered meanings. It can denote alleviation or reduction of affliction, the process of healing or improvement, and even the attenuation or fading of strength. In biblical usage, it may also refer to a spirit of heaviness or weakness that is replaced by restoration. In this context, however, the term is used ironically—Nineveh's wound is beyond *kēhâh*. There will be no softening, no remedy, no reversal.

Ultimately, Nahum's prophecy serves as a sobering reminder that unchecked power and cruelty cannot endure. Divine justice may be delayed, but it is never denied. When the wicked refuse to repent, their fall is not only inevitable—it is profound, public, and total.

Chapter 30
Healing in the book of Malachi

1. Malachi 4:1-3

1 "For behold, the day is coming, Burning like an oven, And all the proud, yes, all who do wickedly will be stubble. And the day which is coming shall burn them up," Says the Lord of hosts, "That will leave them neither root nor branch.

2 But to you who fear My name The Sun of Righteousness shall arise With healing in His wings; And you shall go out And grow fat like stall-fed calves.

3 You shall trample the wicked, For they shall be ashes under the soles of your feet On the day that I do this," Says the Lord of hosts.

Summary

In this profound and prophetic passage from the book of Malachi, the prophet proclaims the coming of the Great Day of the Lord—a day marked by both divine judgment and ultimate restoration. Malachi presents a vivid contrast between the fate of the wicked and the reward of the righteous, offering a sobering warning and a radiant promise. The imagery is striking: God's wrath is likened to a blazing furnace, consuming the arrogant and the evildoers like dry stubble. Their destruction will be absolute, leaving "neither root nor branch"—a metaphor for total eradication, with no hope of renewal or escape.

This judgment is not impulsive or unjust; it is the consequence of persistent rebellion and pride. The proud, who have elevated themselves above God's law, and the wicked, who have perpetuated injustice and oppression, will face the full weight of divine retribution. The furnace symbolizes not only the intensity of God's judgment but also its purifying nature—exposing and eliminating all that is corrupt and ungodly.

In contrast, Malachi offers a message of hope and restoration to those who "fear the Lord"—those who live in reverence, obedience, and faithfulness. For them, "the Sun of Righteousness will rise with healing in its wings." This poetic image evokes warmth, light, and renewal. The sun, as the source of life and growth, becomes a symbol of divine favor and the dawning of a new era. The phrase "healing in its wings" suggests a comprehensive restoration—physical, emotional, and spiritual. It is a promise of wholeness and peace for those who have remained steadfast in their devotion.

In Christian theology, the "Sun of Righteousness" is widely interpreted as a messianic reference to Jesus Christ. This imagery is echoed in Luke 1:78–79, where Zechariah speaks of the coming Messiah as the rising sun who will shine on those living in darkness and guide their feet into the path of peace. Malachi's prophecy thus anticipates the arrival of Christ, who brings salvation, healing, and the fulfillment of God's redemptive plan.

On the Day of the Lord, the righteous will not only be healed—they will flourish. Malachi describes them as leaping like calves released from the stall, a vivid picture of exuberant joy, freedom, and abundance. Their vindication will be evident, and their prosperity unmistakable. In contrast, the wicked—once powerful and oppressive—will be reduced to ashes under the feet of the righteous. This reversal of fortunes underscores the justice of God: the humbled will be exalted, and the exalted will be brought low.

This passage reveals three central theological themes:

- **The Dual Nature of the Day of the Lord**: For the wicked, it will be a day of judgment and destruction. For the righteous, it will be a day of joy, liberation, and renewal. The same event yields radically different outcomes depending on one's relationship with God.

- **Messianic Hope**: The "Sun of Righteousness" heralds the coming of Christ, who brings healing and redemption. His arrival fulfills God's promise to restore His people and conquer evil.

- **Divine Justice**: Malachi affirms that God does not ignore wickedness. His justice is both retributive and redemptive—punishing evil while lifting up the faithful and healing the broken.

Ultimately, Malachi's prophecy is both a solemn warning and a gracious invitation. It calls readers to examine their hearts, turn from pride and injustice, and embrace the fear of the Lord. In doing so, they will find healing, joy, and eternal restoration in the light of the coming King.

The Hebrew word translated as "healing" is *marpe*, meaning cure, remedy, or health. It encompasses physical, emotional, and spiritual well-being, pointing to the holistic restoration promised to those who walk in reverence before God.

PART 6

HEALTH IN THE OLD TESTAMENT

Chapter 31
Health in the book of Genesis

1. Genesis 43:26-28

26 And when Joseph came home, they brought him the present which was in their hand into the house, and bowed down before him to the earth.

27 Then he asked them about their well-being, and said, "Is your father well, the old man of whom you spoke? Is he still alive?"

28 And they answered, "Your servant our father is in good health; he is still alive." And they bowed their heads down and prostrated themselves.

Summary

In this deeply moving passage from the Book of Genesis, Joseph's brothers are brought to his residence during their second journey to Egypt. Still unaware of his true identity, they approach him with gifts and bow low before him in reverence. This moment marks a significant turning point in the narrative, as their gestures of humility and submission fulfill the prophetic dreams Joseph had shared in his youth—visions that once provoked their jealousy and hostility (Genesis 37:5–10). What was once dismissed as youthful arrogance is now realized with divine precision.

Joseph, now a powerful Egyptian official, receives them with composed grace, maintaining the secrecy of his identity. He inquires about the well-being of their elderly father, Jacob, revealing a personal concern that hints at the enduring emotional bond he still feels for his family. The brothers respond that their father is alive and well, despite his age. Overcome with emotion, they bow once more before Joseph, unknowingly reenacting the very dream they had once scorned. This scene is rich with theological and relational significance, offering insight into God's providence, human transformation, and the slow unfolding of reconciliation.

- **Fulfillment of Prophetic Vision:** The brothers' repeated acts of reverence toward Joseph serve as the direct fulfillment of the dreams he received in his youth. What once seemed implausible or self-serving is now revealed as a divinely orchestrated reality. This fulfillment affirms that God's purposes are not thwarted by human opposition. Despite betrayal, suffering, and long delays, God's sovereign plan unfolds with perfect timing. Joseph's elevation and his brothers' submission are not merely political developments—they are spiritual confirmations of divine intent.

- **Joseph's Concealment and Discernment:** Joseph's decision to withhold his identity is not rooted in bitterness or revenge, but in wisdom and discernment. Through a series of carefully crafted interactions, he tests his brothers' character, seeking evidence of repentance and transformation. His restraint demonstrates emotional maturity and spiritual insight. Rather than rushing into reconciliation, Joseph allows time and circumstance to reveal whether trust can be reestablished. His approach underscores the importance of discernment in the process of healing fractured relationships.

- **The Seeds of Reconciliation:** Though Joseph has not yet revealed himself, his inquiries about Jacob and his attentiveness to his brothers' responses suggest a deep longing for reconnection. His concern for his father and his careful observation of his brothers' behavior indicate that, beneath the surface, his heart remains tethered to his family. This moment plants the seeds of reconciliation, foreshadowing a future reunion that will restore not only familial ties but also fractured identities and broken trust.

In sum, this passage is layered with emotional and spiritual depth. It captures the delicate tension between concealment and revelation, justice and mercy, prophecy and fulfillment. Joseph's journey from dreamer to ruler, and his brothers' transformation from betrayers to humbled men, converge in a scene that prepares the way for healing and restoration. It reminds us that even in seasons of uncertainty and trial, God is weaving a redemptive narrative—one that honors truth, invites repentance, and ultimately restores what has been lost.

The word translated as "health" in this passage is rooted in the Hebrew phrase *shalom shalom*, which literally means "peace, peace." This repetition intensifies the meaning, conveying not just the absence of conflict but the presence of total wholeness—a life in harmony with God, others, and oneself. It signifies a state of complete well-being, where every need is met and every relationship is rightly ordered. In the context of Joseph's story, *shalom shalom* anticipates the peace that will soon emerge from years of pain, separation, and divine preparation.

Chapter 32
Health in the book of Samuel

1. 2 Samuel 20:8-10

8 When they were at the large stone which is in Gibeon, Amasa came before them. Now Joab was dressed in battle armor; on it was a belt with a sword fastened in its sheath at his hips; and as he was going forward, it fell out.

9 Then Joab said to Amasa, "Are you in health, my brother?" And Joab took Amasa by the beard with his right hand to kiss him.

10 But Amasa did not notice the sword that was in Joab's hand. And he struck him with it in the stomach, and his entrails poured out on the ground; and he did not strike him again. Thus he died.

Then Joab and Abishai his brother pursued Sheba the son of Bichri.

Summary

This passage recounts the brutal and calculated assassination of Amasa by Joab, a moment that underscores the treacherous undercurrents of political and military leadership during King David's reign. Amasa, having been entrusted by David with the task of rallying the men of Judah in preparation for a campaign against Sheba—a rebel who had risen against the king—was returning from his mission when he encountered Joab. Joab, accompanied by Abishai and their troops, was also en route under David's command to suppress Sheba's insurrection.

Upon meeting Amasa, Joab greets him with apparent warmth and familiarity, saying, "Are you well, my brother?" This greeting, however, masks a deadly intent. In a gesture that mimics affection, Joab reaches out with his right hand, grasping Amasa by the beard as if to kiss him—a customary sign of respect and kinship. In that moment of vulnerability, Joab draws his sword and strikes Amasa in the abdomen, killing him instantly and spilling his entrails onto the ground. Without remorse or hesitation, Joab, Abishai, and their forces continue on their way, leaving Amasa's lifeless body by the roadside.

This act of treachery is particularly chilling given the context and the symbolic weight of Joab's greeting. The phrase "Are you well?" is translated from the Hebrew expression *shâlôm shâlôm*, a repetition that intensifies the meaning of *shâlôm*, which encompasses peace, wholeness, and well-being. In ancient Hebrew culture, repeating the word conveyed a deep and sincere blessing—an invocation of health, prosperity, and divine favor. Joab's use of this phrase, moments before committing murder, adds a layer of bitter irony and underscores the depth of his deception.

Several key themes emerge from this passage:

- **Betrayal and Violence**: Joab's actions reveal a ruthless willingness to eliminate perceived threats to his authority. Despite Amasa's loyalty to David and his role in the king's command structure, Joab views him as a rival and disposes of him through deceit and violence. This moment reflects the volatile nature of leadership and the lengths to which individuals may go to preserve power.

- **The Corruption of Peaceful Symbols**: The use of *shâlôm shâlôm*—a phrase rich in spiritual and cultural significance—juxtaposed with an act of murder, highlights the distortion of sacred language for manipulative ends. Joab weaponizes a blessing, turning a gesture of peace into a prelude to death.

- **Political Intrigue and Moral Complexity**: This episode illustrates the moral ambiguity that often accompanies political maneuvering in Scripture. Joab, though a loyal servant of David in many respects, repeatedly acts outside the bounds of justice, raising questions about loyalty, ambition, and the cost of unchecked authority.

In sum, the murder of Amasa is not merely a historical footnote—it is a vivid portrayal of betrayal cloaked in civility, and a stark reminder of the dangers that arise when power is pursued without integrity.

Chapter 33
Health in the book of Psalms

1. Psalms 42:9-11 (KJV)

9 I will say unto God my rock, Why hast thou forgotten me? why go I mourning because of the oppression of the enemy?

10 As with a sword in my bones, mine enemies reproach me; while they say daily unto me, Where is thy God?

11 Why art thou cast down, O my soul? and why art thou disquieted within me? hope thou in God: for I shall yet praise him, who is the health of my countenance, and my God.

Summary

This passage from the Psalms, written by the sons of Korah, paints a powerful picture of deep emotional pain and spiritual struggle. The writer is overwhelmed by suffering and the cruel words of his enemies. In his distress, he speaks openly to God, asking hard questions: "Why have you forgotten me? Why must I go about mourning, oppressed by the enemy?" These words show not only physical hardship but also a strong feeling of being abandoned and spiritually lost.

The psalmist's enemies make things worse by mocking his faith. They ask, "Where is your God?" Their words cut deep, shaking the foundation of his trust in God's presence. In this moment of emotional collapse, the psalmist does something remarkable—he speaks to his own soul. "Why are you downcast, my soul? Why so disturbed within me?" This inner conversation shows the tension between what he believes and what he feels. His faith tells him to trust, but his emotions are heavy with sorrow.

Instead of giving in to despair, he chooses to hope. He tells his soul to keep trusting in God and promises to continue praising Him. He declares that God is "the salvation of my face and my God." This statement doesn't come from a place of comfort or rescue—it comes from a decision to believe, even when things look bleak. It's a choice to trust in God's character, even when there's no visible sign of help.

This passage teaches several important spiritual lessons:

- **Honest Prayer**

    The psalmist shows us that it's okay to be honest with God. He doesn't hide his pain or pretend everything is fine. He brings his sorrow, confusion, and questions directly to God. This kind of prayer is real and raw. It reminds us that God welcomes our true feelings and can handle our deepest struggles.

- **The Battle Between Mind and Soul**

  There's a clear difference between the psalmist's thoughts and his emotions. His mind remembers God's truth and urges his soul to rise above despair. But his soul is weighed down by fear and sadness. Many believers know this struggle—trying to hold on to faith while feeling overwhelmed. The psalmist doesn't ignore his feelings. Instead, he speaks truth to them, guiding his soul toward hope.

- **Choosing Hope in Darkness**

  One of the strongest themes in this passage is the psalmist's decision to hope. Even when surrounded by pain and mockery, he remembers God's past faithfulness. That memory becomes his anchor. He praises God, not because everything is fixed, but because he trusts that God will act. This shows that hope isn't based on circumstances—it's rooted in who God is.

This psalm is a powerful example of how faith can survive in hard times. It doesn't deny suffering but faces it with courage. Through honest prayer, self-reflection, and a firm choice to hope, the psalmist shows us how to walk through despair without being defeated by it. His words invite us to speak truth to our own troubled hearts, to remember God's goodness, and to keep praising Him—even when life is painful.

The word "health" in this passage comes from the Hebrew word *Yeshua*, which means "salvation" or "God saves." This word appears often in Scripture and is used in the New Testament to refer to Jesus. But it's more than just a name—it carries deep meaning. *Yeshua* speaks of God's help, His power to rescue, and His love that heals and restores. It points to complete salvation: healing for the heart, peace for the soul, and a renewed relationship with God. In this psalm, the psalmist clings to *Yeshua*—to the hope that God will save, restore, and bring peace, even in the darkest moments.

2. Psalms 43:5 (KJV)

5 Why art thou cast down, O my soul? and why art thou disquieted within me? hope in God: for I shall yet praise him, who is the health of my countenance, and my God.

Summary

This passage from the Psalms offers a heartfelt and honest look at someone struggling with deep emotional and spiritual pain. The psalmist is facing both inner sadness and outer trouble. In response, he speaks directly to his own soul: "Why are you cast down, O my soul? Why are you disquieted within me?" These words show that he is aware of the gap between what he believes about God and what he feels in the moment—a tension many people experience during hard times.

Instead of letting despair take over, the psalmist makes a clear and intentional choice. He tells his soul to hope in God and declares that he will praise the Lord again. This is not just wishful thinking—it is a strong act of faith. Even though his situation hasn't changed, he chooses to trust in God's goodness and promises. His decision shows spiritual maturity: he refuses to let emotions control him and instead holds on to what he knows is true about God.

He describes God as "the health of my countenance and my God." The word "health" here comes from the Hebrew word *Yeshua*, which means "salvation" or "God saves." This word is deeply important in the Bible and is often used in the New Testament to refer to Jesus. But *Yeshua* is more than a name—it represents God's power to rescue, heal, and restore. It speaks of complete salvation: healing for the heart, peace for the soul, and a renewed relationship with God.

When the psalmist uses this word, he is not just talking about feeling better or being safe. He is declaring his trust in God's ability to save and restore. By calling God his *Yeshua*, he is saying that his hope is in the One who brings light into darkness and turns sorrow into joy.

This passage teaches two important spiritual lessons:

- **Active Faith**: The psalmist's words show that faith is a choice. It's not just a feeling that comes and goes—it's something we decide to hold on to. Even when life is hard and answers are unclear, we can speak truth to ourselves and choose to trust in God's promises.

- **Hope for Future Praise**: The psalmist believes that his pain will not last forever. He looks forward to the day when he will praise God again. His grief becomes the ground where hope grows. This kind of faith turns sadness into expectation and prepares the heart for joy.

In the end, this passage reminds us that faith often grows strongest in hard times. It encourages us to speak truth to our own hearts, to trust in God's saving power, and to believe that sorrow will one day be replaced with praise. *Yeshua*—God who saves—is our hope, our healing, and our peace.

3. Psalms 67:1-2 (KJV)

1 God be merciful unto us, and bless us; and cause his face to shine upon us; Selah.

2 That thy way may be known upon earth, thy saving health among all nations.

Summary

This passage from the Psalms is a heartfelt prayer asking God for grace and blessing—not just for His people, but for the whole world. The psalmist is not only thinking about personal or national needs. He is asking that God's ways, His saving power, and His goodness be known among all nations. His prayer reaches beyond borders and cultures, showing a deep desire for everyone to know and worship the one true God.

At the center of this prayer is a longing for God's salvation to be seen everywhere. The psalmist hopes that the physical and spiritual rescue experienced by Israel will become a witness to others. He wants the story of God's help to inspire people from every nation to turn to Him. This vision is not limited—it looks forward to a time when God's mercy and justice will bring people together in praise.

The word "health" in this passage carries deep meaning. In Hebrew, the word used is *Yeshua*, which means "He saves" or "salvation." It comes from the root word *yasha*, meaning "to rescue" or "to deliver." So when the psalmist speaks of health, he is not just talking about feeling better physically. He is declaring that God is the one who saves and restores. *Yeshua* is a word full of hope—it speaks of God stepping in to help, heal, and bring people back to Himself.

In the bigger story of the Bible, *Yeshua* becomes more than just a word. It is the name given to Jesus. The name Jesus is the Greek form of *Yeshua*, and it shows that Jesus is the fulfillment of this ancient hope. Through Him, the salvation promised to Israel is now offered to everyone. The psalmist's prayer, though written long before Jesus came, points forward to the day when God's rescue would be available to all people through Christ.

This passage teaches two important lessons:

- **Blessing as a Witness**: The psalmist knows that when God blesses His people, it's not just for them. It's meant to show others who God is. When people see God's kindness, they are drawn to Him. Blessing becomes a way to share God's love and power with the world.

- **Hope for All Nations**: The psalmist hopes that God's saving work will reach beyond Israel to every nation. This hope is fulfilled in Jesus, who brings salvation to all. The use of *Yeshua* connects the Old Testament promise with the New Testament reality, showing that God's plan is for everyone.

In short, this psalm is a prayer that starts with personal need and grows into a global vision. It reminds us that God's blessings are meant to reveal His glory. Through *Yeshua*, we see God's heart—a heart that wants to save, heal, and bring all people into worship and peace.

Chapter 34
Health in the book of Proverbs

1. Proverbs 3:5-8

5 Trust in the Lord with all your heart, And lean not on your own understanding;

6 In all your ways acknowledge Him, And He shall direct your paths.

7 Do not be wise in your own eyes; Fear the Lord and depart from evil.

8 It will be health to your flesh, And strength to your bones.

Summary

This passage from the book of Proverbs shares timeless wisdom from King Solomon to his son, offering spiritual guidance that still speaks clearly today. Solomon encourages his son to trust the Lord completely, reminding him that true wisdom doesn't come from human thinking but from God's direction. He warns against relying only on personal understanding and urges him to acknowledge God in every part of life—decisions, actions, and intentions.

When we do this, God promises to guide us, making our paths straight and filled with purpose.

Solomon's words call for full surrender. Instead of depending on ourselves, we are invited to depend on God. This kind of humility doesn't mean giving up responsibility—it means recognizing that God's wisdom is greater than ours and trusting Him to lead us. When we let go of control and lean on God, we gain spiritual clarity and peace.

He also teaches his son to fear the Lord and turn away from evil. This fear isn't about being afraid—it's about having deep respect, awe, and a desire to obey. When we truly honor God, we naturally want to avoid what is wrong and live in a way that pleases Him. This reverence shapes our character and helps us walk in righteousness.

The passage ends with a powerful promise: living this way will bring health to the body and strength to the bones. The Hebrew word used for "health" is *riphuth*, which comes from the verb *rapha*, meaning "to heal" or "to restore." This word goes beyond physical wellness—it speaks of full restoration of body, mind, and spirit. Solomon is saying that when we live in harmony with God, we experience true wholeness. Our inner peace and physical strength are connected to our spiritual posture.

This passage highlights three key spiritual truths:

- **Complete Trust in God**: Solomon teaches that trusting God fully is the beginning of wisdom. It means letting go of our own plans and believing that God's way is better. This kind of trust brings peace and direction.

- **God's Guidance in Our Lives**: When we invite God into every part of our lives, He promises to guide us. His guidance isn't just about decisions—it's about living with purpose and walking in step with His will.

- **Healing Through Reverence and Obedience**: Respecting God and turning away from evil leads to healing. Solomon connects spiritual devotion with physical and emotional health. The word *riphuth* reminds us that God's healing reaches every part of who we are.

In short, Solomon's advice offers a path to wisdom, peace, and restoration. It invites us to trust God deeply, live humbly, and walk in obedience. Through this, we find not only spiritual strength but complete healing—a wellness that flows from a life aligned with God.

2. Proverbs 4:20-22

20 My son, give attention to my words; Incline your ear to my sayings.

21 Do not let them depart from your eyes; Keep them in the midst of your heart;

22 For they are life to those who find them, And health to all their flesh.

Summary

In this passage from the book of Proverbs, King Solomon offers wise and heartfelt advice to his son, encouraging him to fully embrace the teachings that come from God. Solomon's words are not just about gaining knowledge—they are deeply spiritual and practical. He urges his son to listen carefully, to hold these teachings close, and to keep them in his heart. These instructions are meant to guide his life, not just for a moment, but as lasting truths to live by.

Solomon explains that those who find and hold onto this wisdom will experience both life and health. The word "health" here is translated from the Hebrew word *marpê*, which carries a rich and layered meaning. It goes far beyond physical wellness. *Marpê* speaks to the healing and restoring power of wisdom—its ability to bring peace, strength, and wholeness to every part of life.

The meaning of *marpê* includes several important ideas:

- **Healing and Treatment**: At its most basic level, *marpê* refers to physical healing. It suggests that wisdom can act like medicine, helping the body recover and grow stronger.

- **Overall Well-being**: *Marpê* also points to complete wellness. It includes mental clarity, emotional balance, and spiritual peace. It describes a life that is healthy in every way.

- **Remedy or Cure**: The word can also mean a specific solution or treatment that brings relief. In this sense, wisdom is like a divine prescription for the problems and pains of life.

- **Peace and Calm**: Figuratively, *marpê* evokes a sense of calm and serenity. It can describe a gentle presence or a peaceful attitude—something that brings harmony to relationships and quiet strength to the soul.

Solomon's teaching shows that divine wisdom is holistic. It's not just about knowing right from wrong—it affects every part of who we are. When we live by God's wisdom, we experience strength in our bodies, clarity in our minds, and peace in our hearts. The connection between spiritual truth and physical health is real and meaningful. The Bible often shows that body, mind, and spirit are connected, and that healing in one area can bring healing to others.

This passage reminds us of the power of God's Word. Solomon presents wisdom as something alive—something that feeds us, heals us, and helps us grow. His advice is both urgent and loving, showing that following God's instruction leads to a full and flourishing life.

In short, Solomon's counsel is a call to live wisely and fully. It invites us to treat God's Word not just as information, but as life-giving truth. When we treasure divine wisdom and let it shape how we think, speak, and act, we open ourselves to God's healing work—*marpê*—in every part of our lives.

3. Proverbs 12:18

18 There is one who speaks like the piercings of a sword, But the tongue of the wise promotes health.

Summary

In this passage from the book of Proverbs, King Solomon offers powerful wisdom about the importance of how we speak. He compares two kinds of people—those who use their words carelessly and those who speak with wisdom. Solomon says that reckless words are like swords, cutting and hurting others. But wise speech brings healing, comfort, and peace to those who hear it.

The Hebrew word translated as "health" in this verse is *marpê*, which carries deep meaning. It comes from the root word *rapha*, meaning "to heal" or "to restore." *Marpê* refers not only to physical healing but also to emotional, relational, and spiritual well-being. It describes the kind of healing that touches every part of life—body, mind, and soul.

Marpê can mean:

- **Physical Healing**: It suggests that wise words can help restore strength and bring relief, much like medicine for the body.
- **Complete Wellness**: It includes peace of mind, emotional balance, and spiritual calm.

It's about feeling whole and well in every area of life.

- **A Remedy or Cure**: Wise speech acts like a treatment for the wounds of life. It brings comfort and helps people recover from pain.

- **Peace and Serenity**: *Marpê* also points to a gentle and calming presence. Words that are kind and thoughtful can bring peace to tense situations and restore broken relationships.

Solomon's teaching shows that words are never neutral. They have the power to shape lives, influence hearts, and change outcomes. As Proverbs 18:21 says, "Death and life are in the power of the tongue." Words can build up or tear down, encourage or discourage, heal or harm. Though small, the tongue has great influence, and how we use it matters deeply.

This passage also shows the difference between wise and foolish people. Wise individuals understand the impact of their words. They speak with care, kindness, and purpose. Their words bring healing and hope. Foolish people, on the other hand, speak without thinking. Their words often come from pride, anger, or ignorance, and they can cause lasting damage.

James 3:5–10 supports this idea, warning that the tongue can be dangerous if not controlled. It can stir up conflict, damage relationships, and spread harm. That's why Solomon's advice is so important—it's a call to be intentional and careful with our speech.

In the end, Solomon urges us to use our words wisely. Speech is not just about communication—it reflects what's in our hearts. When guided by wisdom and humility, our words can bring *marpê*—true healing—to others. When misused, they can cause deep wounds.

This passage invites us to speak in ways that reflect God's love and character. By choosing words that heal, encourage, and restore, we become part of God's work in bringing peace and wholeness to a hurting world.

4. Proverbs 13:17

17 A wicked messenger falls into trouble, But a faithful ambassador brings health.

Summary

In this passage from the book of Proverbs, Solomon offers wise insight into the power of communication and the importance of integrity. He compares two types of messengers—one who is faithful and brings healing, and another who is unreliable and causes harm. This contrast goes beyond personal behavior; it speaks to leadership, trust, and the well-being of entire communities.

The faithful messenger is described as someone who brings "health," a word translated from the Hebrew *marpê*. This term, rooted in the verb *rapha*, meaning "to heal" or "to restore," carries deep and layered meaning. While it can refer to physical healing, *marpê* also speaks to emotional, relational, and even national restoration. It represents a kind of wholeness that touches every part of life.

Depending on the context, *marpê* can mean:

- **Healing**: The process of restoring strength and wellness, whether in the body or in the heart.
- **Health**: A general sense of well-being, including mental and emotional stability.
- **Medicine**: A remedy or treatment that brings relief and recovery.
- **Peacefulness**: A calm and steady spirit that brings comfort and stability.
- **Deliverance**: Rescue or relief from trouble, especially in times of crisis or confusion.

In this passage, *marpê* is best understood as deliverance. The faithful messenger is not just someone who speaks truthfully—he is someone who brings clarity, peace, and resolution. His reliability helps restore trust and stability in the community or nation he serves. On the other hand, the unfaithful messenger—someone who misleads, delays, or distorts the truth—creates confusion and can cause serious harm. His actions may lead to broken relationships, poor decisions, or even conflict.

The word "messenger" or "ambassador" adds a broader meaning to the text. In ancient times, messengers often carried important news between leaders or nations. Their honesty and accuracy could shape the outcome of political decisions, military actions, or community plans. A faithful messenger was a source of *marpê*—healing and peace—while an unreliable one could bring disaster.

Solomon's teaching highlights the power of words and the importance of character. When truth is spoken with integrity, it brings healing and unity. But when words are twisted or misused, they can divide and damage. This wisdom applies not only to leaders and diplomats but to everyday life. In families, workplaces, and friendships, being a trustworthy communicator means sharing truth with kindness and clarity.

This passage invites us to think about how we represent truth in our own lives. Whether we're leading others, offering support, or simply sharing information, we are called to be faithful messengers. By speaking with honesty and compassion, we become channels of *marpê*—bringing healing, peace, and restoration wherever we go.

5. Proverbs 16:23-24

23 The heart of the wise teaches his mouth, And adds learning to his lips.

24 Pleasant words are like a honeycomb, Sweetness to the soul and health to the bones.

Summary

In this passage from the book of Proverbs, Solomon offers deep and practical wisdom about the power of speech. He focuses on the kind of words that come from a wise heart—words that do more than inform or impress. They bring comfort, clarity, and healing. Solomon compares these words to honey, a powerful image that speaks to both sweetness and nourishment. Just as honey was treasured in ancient times for its taste and healing properties, wise speech is valued for its ability to soothe and restore.

Solomon's metaphor is rich with meaning. Honey was not only a delicacy but also a symbol of purity and natural healing. By likening wise words to honey, Solomon shows that speech can be both pleasant and powerful. Words from a wise person do not stir up conflict or confusion. Instead, they calm the heart, guide the mind, and refresh the soul. They are gentle and thoughtful, offering peace to those who are weary and direction to those who feel lost.

The word "health" in this passage is translated from the Hebrew word *marpê*, which appears several times in Solomon's writings. *Marpê* comes from the verb *rapha*, meaning "to heal," "to restore," or "to repair." While it often refers to physical healing, its meaning goes much deeper. In biblical usage, *marpê* can describe emotional relief, spiritual peace, and even a calm and steady spirit. It is a word that speaks to full and balanced well-being.

In this context, *marpê* is not just about physical health. It points to a kind of inner peace that comes from wise and gentle speech. The words of the wise are like medicine—not only for the body, but for the heart and mind. They help people feel safe, understood, and supported. Solomon's use of *marpê* shows that true wisdom brings healing in every area of life.

This passage teaches several important lessons:

- **The Source of Wise Speech.** Solomon reminds us that speech reflects the condition of the heart. Words are not random—they come from within. Jesus echoes this in Luke 6:45:

  "... for of the abundance of the heart his mouth speaketh."

- **What we say reveals who we are.** A wise person speaks with kindness and truth because their heart is shaped by God's wisdom. Their words are not just clever—they are sincere and life-giving.

- **The Power of Words.** Words can build up or tear down. Solomon's description of wise speech as sweet and healing matches Paul's teaching in Ephesians 4:29:

  "Let no corrupt communication proceed out of your mouth, but that which is good to the use of edifying, that it may minister grace unto the hearers."

  Thoughtful words can mend broken hearts, encourage the discouraged, and bring peace to tense situations. In a world full of harsh voices, speaking with grace is a powerful gift.

- **The Holistic Effect of Wisdom.** Solomon's use of marpê encourages us to see the full impact of wise speech. It doesn't just help people think better—it helps them feel better and live better. Wise words promote spiritual strength, emotional balance, and even physical health. This reflects the biblical view that body, mind, and spirit are connected. When we speak with love and truth, we help others experience healing in every part of their lives.

- **The Call to Grow in Wisdom.** This passage is also a call to develop inner wisdom. Solomon urges us to care for our hearts, knowing that what's inside will shape what comes out. This means spending time in prayer, reading Scripture, and practicing humility. As we grow in wisdom, our words will naturally reflect God's love and truth. Our speech will become a source of marpê— bringing healing and peace to those around us.

Solomon's message is still relevant today. In a time when words are shared quickly and often without thought, his wisdom invites us to slow down and consider what we say. Are our words like honey— sweet, healing, and life-giving? Do they offer *marpê* to those who hear them? This passage challenges us to speak with purpose, compassion, and depth. When we do, we reflect God's heart and become part of His work of restoration in the world.

Chapter 35
Health in the book of Isaiah

1. Isaiah 58:5-8 (KJV)

5 Is it such a fast that I have chosen? a day for a man to afflict his soul? is it to bow down his head as a bulrush, and to spread sackcloth and ashes under him? wilt thou call this a fast, and an acceptable day to the Lord?

6 Is not this the fast that I have chosen? to loose the bands of wickedness, to undo the heavy burdens, and to let the oppressed go free, and that ye break every yoke?

7 Is it not to deal thy bread to the hungry, and that thou bring the poor that are cast out to thy house? when thou seest the naked, that thou cover him; and that thou hide not thyself from thine own flesh?

8 Then shall thy light break forth as the morning, and thine health shall spring forth speedily: and thy righteousness shall go before thee; the glory of the Lord shall be thy reward.

Summary

In this powerful passage from the book of Isaiah, God instructs the prophet to raise his voice like a trumpet in response to the cries of the people of Israel. The people are confused and discouraged. They have fasted, mourned, and practiced outward signs of humility, yet they feel ignored by God. They ask why their spiritual efforts seem to go unnoticed. Through Isaiah, God answers with clarity and conviction: their fasting is empty because it is rooted in selfishness, conflict, and injustice.

Instead of drawing closer to God, their fasts have become occasions for division and harm. They argue, exploit others, and act violently—all while appearing religious. God exposes the gap between their rituals and their behavior. He makes it clear that He does not delight in outward signs of humility—bowing the head, wearing sackcloth, or sitting in ashes—when those actions are not matched by compassion and righteousness. These traditions, though familiar, are meaningless without a heart that reflects God's love and justice.

God then reveals the kind of fast He truly desires. It is not about self-denial alone, but about transforming lives and communities. The fast God chooses is one that breaks chains of injustice, lifts burdens, and sets people free. It is a fast that feeds the hungry, shelters the homeless, and clothes those in need. This kind of fasting is not just spiritual—it is practical, active, and deeply rooted in mercy. It reflects God's heart and calls His people to live out their faith through love and generosity.

When this kind of fast is embraced, God promises powerful blessings. "Then your light will break forth like the dawn," He says, "and your healing will spring up quickly." The word "healing" here is translated from the Hebrew word *arukah*, which carries rich meaning. Derived from a root that suggests length and completeness, *arukah* refers to full restoration—health, wholeness, and renewal. It is not a quick fix or surface-level cure. It describes a deep, lasting process of being made whole again.

In Scripture, *arukah* is often used to describe something that has been returned to its proper state—mended, perfected, and restored. It speaks to physical healing, but also to emotional, spiritual, and relational renewal. When people live in alignment with God's ways—pursuing justice, showing mercy, and walking with integrity—they open themselves to this kind of healing. Their lives become marked by peace, strength, and divine favor. Their righteousness leads the way, and God's presence protects and surrounds them.

This passage highlights two key truths:

- **Worship Must Include Justice.** Isaiah's message challenges the idea that religious rituals alone can please God. While spiritual practices are important, they are not enough if they are disconnected from ethical living. Some may think that attending worship or fasting excuses them from caring for others, or that doing good deeds replaces the need for spiritual devotion. But Scripture shows that both are essential. The story of Eli and his sons, Hophni and Phinehas (1 Samuel 2:12–36), is a clear warning. Though they held religious authority, they abused their roles and dishonored God. Their failure to live righteously led to judgment. Isaiah's words remind us that God cares about both our worship and our actions. True devotion means honoring God in the temple and in daily life. It means combining reverence with compassion.

- **Holistic Blessing Through Obedience.** When believers follow the fast God desires—one marked by justice, mercy, and generosity—they receive arukah, the blessing of full restoration. This healing is not temporary or shallow. It is deep, lasting, and touches every part of life—body, soul, relationships, and community. It is the kind of wholeness that only God can give, and it flows from a life lived in harmony with His will.

This passage invites us to reflect on our spiritual practices. Are they just routines, or do they reflect God's heart? Do they lead to real change in our lives and in the world around us? Isaiah's message calls us to a fast that goes beyond giving something up—it is a fast that gives to others, lifts the oppressed, and shows God's love in action.

In the end, God is not asking for empty gestures. He is calling His people to live out His character. When they do, their lives shine with light, their healing springs forth, and their righteousness opens the way for divine blessing. The glory of the Lord surrounds them, and they walk in the fullness of *arukah*—a life restored, renewed, and made whole by the hand of God.

Chapter 36
Health in the book of Jeremiah

1. Jeremiah 8:13-15

13 "I will surely consume them," says the Lord. "No grapes shall be on the vine, Nor figs on the fig tree, And the leaf shall fade; And the things I have given them shall pass away from them." ' "

14 "Why do we sit still? Assemble yourselves, And let us enter the fortified cities, And let us be silent there. For the Lord our God has put us to silence And given us water of gall to drink, Because we have sinned against the Lord.

15 "We looked for peace, but no good came; And for a time of health, and there was trouble!

Summary

This sobering passage from the book of Jeremiah offers a vivid picture of divine judgment against the kingdom of Judah—a direct result of long-standing sin and spiritual rebellion. Speaking through the prophet, God announces His decision to bring devastation upon the land and its people. Both leaders and citizens are held accountable for abandoning truth, corrupting worship, and breaking the covenant God had entrusted to them.

God's judgment is not random or harsh without reason. It is rooted in justice. The leaders, who were supposed to guide the people in righteousness, instead led them into deception. Their teachings were not based on God's truth, and their actions showed a clear disregard for His commands. Because of this, God chose to bring consequences—not just spiritual separation, but real, visible destruction. One of the most striking signs of this judgment was the collapse of agriculture. The land, once a symbol of God's blessing and provision, would be stripped bare. Crops would fail, food would disappear, and the gifts God had generously provided would be taken away.

This loss was not only physical—it carried deep symbolic meaning. In ancient Israel, agriculture was more than an economic system. It was a sign of God's favor and covenant. When the harvest disappeared, it showed that the relationship between God and His people had been broken. It was a painful, public reminder that divine blessing had been withdrawn.

Faced with this disaster, the people of Judah did not respond with repentance or humility. Instead of turning to God and asking for mercy, they withdrew. They gathered in fortified cities, choosing silence over reconciliation. Their words reveal a tragic sense of defeat: "The Lord has silenced us and made us drink poisoned water because of our sins against Him." This statement admits guilt, but it lacks the kind of sorrow that leads to change. It is a confession without hope—a recognition of God's anger without a desire for healing.

The people had longed for peace, but it never came. They had hoped for healing, but instead found only suffering. The word "health" in this passage is translated from the Hebrew word *marpê*, which means healing, restoration, and wholeness. It comes from the verb *rapha*, meaning "to heal" or "to repair." *Marpê* often refers to a process of renewal—whether physical, emotional, or spiritual. But in this passage, *marpê* is noticeably absent. What should have been a time of healing became a time of pain. The people expected God to intervene, but instead they experienced silence and judgment.

This passage highlights two important spiritual truths:

- **Divine Justice.** God's judgment on Judah was a direct result of their sin. His justice is not unpredictable—it reflects His character and His covenant. As Paul writes in Galatians 6:7, **"Whatever a man sows, that he will also reap."** Judah had sown rebellion, lies, and spiritual neglect. They reaped destruction, silence, and loss. The damage was complete: spiritual distance from God, collapse of the land's productivity, and national decline. This shows how seriously God views covenant disobedience.

    But God's justice is not only about punishment—it is also meant to correct. His judgments are meant to wake people up, to confront them, and to invite them back to Him. In this case, however, the people did not respond. Their retreat into silence and fortified cities showed that they were not willing to return to God. They admitted their guilt but did not ask for forgiveness. The absence of *marpê*—healing—was not because God refused to heal, but because the people refused to repent.

- **The Danger of Hardened Hearts.** Judah's situation shows the danger of hearts that refuse to change. Without true repentance, judgment is not only certain—it becomes final. The people's sorrow was real, but it lacked the humility and brokenness needed for reconciliation. They knew they had sinned, but they did not turn away from it. They suffered the consequences, but they did not seek transformation. This spiritual stagnation made it impossible for them to receive the healing they needed.

The silence they experienced was not just about circumstances—it was spiritual. God had withdrawn His voice, His favor, and His healing presence. The poisoned water they drank symbolized their inner condition: bitter, toxic, and lifeless. They had hoped for peace, but found conflict. They had longed for healing, but were met with despair.

This passage is a serious reminder of the weight of sin and the importance of repentance. It shows the painful results of ignoring God and the emptiness of religious rituals without a real relationship with Him. But it also points to a hopeful truth: *marpê*—healing—is always possible when people truly turn to God. His justice is real, but so is His mercy. The tragedy of Judah was not that God refused to heal, but that the people refused to seek Him.

Their story invites us to respond differently. Instead of retreating into silence or relying on empty rituals, we are called to repent sincerely, live righteously, and embrace the healing God is always ready to give. *Marpê* is not just a word—it is a promise. It speaks of restoration, peace, and wholeness. And it is available to all who turn to God with open hearts.

2. Jeremiah 8:21-22

21 For the hurt of the daughter of my people I am hurt. I am mourning; Astonishment has taken hold of me.

22 Is there no balm in Gilead, Is there no physician there? Why then is there no recovery For the health of the daughter of my people?

Summary

This passage from the book of Jeremiah reveals the deep sorrow and emotional weight carried by the prophet as he intercedes for the people of Judah. Jeremiah is not a distant observer of their suffering—he fully identifies with their pain. Though he remains faithful to God, he chooses to stand with his people in their grief, presenting their brokenness before God with heartfelt urgency.

Jeremiah pleads with God to listen to the cries of a nation overwhelmed by the consequences of its rebellion. In response, God asks a piercing question: "Why have they provoked Me with their carved images and foreign idols?" This question points directly to the heart of Judah's suffering—their persistent idolatry and abandonment of their covenant with God. Instead of worshiping the living God, they have turned to lifeless substitutes, and the result is devastation.

Jeremiah does not try to excuse the people's behavior or soften their guilt. Instead, he turns inward, expressing his own emotional and spiritual pain. He confesses that he is wounded and deeply troubled by the extent of Judah's downfall. His lament is not distant or formal—it is raw and personal. He feels the weight of God's judgment and the sorrow of a land in ruins. His empathy is so complete that he experiences the nation's suffering as if it were his own.

Looking at the destruction around him, Jeremiah asks a haunting question: "Is there no balm in Gilead? Is there no physician there?" These words evoke the image of a place once known for healing—now empty of help. The absence of remedy is not just physical; it is spiritual. The people are wounded in a way that no human medicine can cure. Their condition is beyond natural recovery. Only God's mercy can bring restoration.

The word "health" in this passage is translated from the Hebrew word *arukah*, which means more than just physical healing. It comes from a root that means "to prolong," and it refers to a process of deep, lasting restoration. In Scripture, *arukah* describes something that has been repaired, made whole, and returned to its proper state. It is not a quick fix—it is enduring renewal, a steady flow of divine blessing and vitality.

In this context, the absence of *arukah* reveals a painful truth: Judah has lost access to God's healing presence. Their sins have broken the connection, and the land shows the signs of that separation. The silence, decay, and despair are not random—they are the natural results of spiritual rebellion. Without repentance, the flow of God's blessing is blocked, and the people remain in a state of ruin.

This passage highlights two important themes:

- **Jeremiah's Compassionate Leadership.** Jeremiah's lament shows the heart of a true spiritual leader. Though he has not sinned like the rest of Judah, he does not stand apart in judgment. Instead, he carries their burden and pleads for mercy on their behalf. His deep empathy and sincere prayer reflect the kind of leadership that seeks healing for others, even at personal cost. Jeremiah's identification with his people gives weight to his intercession and shows his commitment to both God and the nation.

- **The Seriousness of Spiritual Illness.** The imagery of wounds and healing points to a deeper reality: sin is a spiritual disease that only God can cure. Judah's idolatry and injustice have left them deeply wounded. The absence of *arukah* is not because God lacks the power to heal—it is because the people refuse to seek His remedy. Healing is available, but it requires a change of heart. Repentance, humility, and a return to God's covenant are the only path to restoration. Until that happens, the wound remains open, and healing remains out of reach.

In conclusion, this passage is a powerful reflection on the cost of turning away from God and the depth of compassion shown by those who intercede. Jeremiah's sorrow invites us to take sin seriously, to recognize the need for repentance, and to believe in the hope of divine restoration. Even in the midst of desolation, the promise of *arukah*—true healing—is still possible. If the people will turn back to God, He is ready to restore what has been broken and bring lasting wholeness.

3. Jeremiah 30:16-17

16 'Therefore all those who devour you shall be devoured; And all your adversaries, every one of them, shall go into captivity; Those who plunder you shall become plunder, And all who prey upon you I will make a prey.

17 For I will restore health to you And heal you of your wounds,' says the Lord, 'Because they called you an outcast saying: "This is Zion; No one seeks her." '

Summary

This passage from the book of Jeremiah delivers a powerful and hopeful message of restoration for Israel and Judah. After a long season of judgment and suffering, God speaks through the prophet to announce that the time of discipline is coming to an end. The nations that had harmed, plundered, and oppressed His people will now face consequences. Those who inflicted pain will experience the same fate they imposed, and the enemies of Israel and Judah will be led into captivity. This reversal is not just political—it reflects God's sovereign justice.

God's promise of restoration is complete and far-reaching. He does not only promise to defend His people; He pledges to heal them. "I will restore your health," He declares, "and I will heal your wounds." This promise goes beyond physical recovery. It includes emotional healing, spiritual renewal, and national restoration. The Hebrew word translated as "health" here is *arukah*, a term rich in meaning and depth.

Arukah comes from the root *arak*, which carries ideas of prolonging, arranging, and enhancing. Its related form, *arek*, often means "long" and is used in phrases like "slow to anger," describing patience and restraint. In this passage, *arukah* refers to a healing process that is intentional, lasting, and complete. It is not a quick fix or surface-level solution. Instead, it speaks of deep restoration—bringing order, strength, and wholeness to what was broken.

The use of *arukah* signals that God's healing is more than physical. It marks the full rehabilitation of His people. It means the return of divine favor, the renewal of identity, and the reestablishment of purpose. The people are not just rescued from danger—they are restored to dignity, reconnected to their calling, and reintegrated into God's plan. *Arukah* is the flow of divine blessing that sets things right and brings lasting peace.

This passage highlights three key spiritual themes:

- **God's Sovereign Justice.** The restoration of Israel and Judah is tied directly to God's justice. The nations that oppressed God's people believed they would escape judgment. But divine justice is never absent—it may be delayed, but it is always sure. God's discipline of His people was not abandonment; it was correction. Now, He turns His attention to their enemies, ensuring that every injustice is answered. This shows that God is not only a healer but also a righteous judge who defends the oppressed.

- **God's Covenant Faithfulness.** Even though Israel and Judah had repeatedly failed, God remained faithful to His covenant. His promises were not canceled by their mistakes. Instead, they were upheld by His unchanging character. The restoration described here is not something the people earned—it is a gift of grace. It reflects God's commitment to His people, even when they stray. This faithfulness offers hope: no matter how far we fall, God's mercy can still bring renewal.

- **Divine Healing and Restoration.** The healing God offers is complete. It touches the soul, the community, and the history of a people. Only God can repair what sin has broken. The word *arukah* reminds us that this healing is a process. It takes time, but it is thorough. It restores what was lost and perfects what was damaged. This restoration is both personal and collective—it renews individuals and rebuilds nations.

In summary, this passage from Jeremiah is a declaration of divine renewal. It assures God's people that their suffering is not the final chapter. Through justice, faithfulness, and healing, God restores dignity, renews purpose, and reestablishes His covenant. The promise of *arukah* invites believers to trust in the steady, powerful work of divine restoration—a process that brings wholeness, peace, and lasting hope to every part of life.

4. Jeremiah 33:4-9

4 "For thus says the Lord, the God of Israel, concerning the houses of this city and the houses of

the kings of Judah, which have been pulled down to fortify against the siege mounds and the sword:

5 'They come to fight with the Chaldeans, but only to fill their places with the dead bodies of men whom I will slay in My anger and My fury, all for whose wickedness I have hidden My face from this city.

6 Behold, I will bring it health and healing; I will heal them and reveal to them the abundance of peace and truth.

7 And I will cause the captives of Judah and the captives of Israel to return, and will rebuild those places as at the first.

8 I will cleanse them from all their iniquity by which they have sinned against Me, and I will pardon all their iniquities by which they have sinned and by which they have transgressed against Me.

9 Then it shall be to Me a name of joy, a praise, and an honor before all nations of the earth, who shall hear all the good that I do to them; they shall fear and tremble for all the goodness and all the prosperity that I provide for it.'

Summary

In the midst of fear, chaos, and the threat of destruction, Jerusalem stands under siege by the powerful Babylonian army. Once a vibrant and sacred city, it is now filled with desperation. Homes are torn down to build defenses, a tragic sign of how daily life has unraveled. In this moment of crisis, God speaks to the prophet Jeremiah with a message that is both sobering and full of hope.

God begins by announcing judgment. The sins of Jerusalem—its corruption, idolatry, and moral failure—have reached a breaking point. The people have turned away from what is right, and now divine justice must be carried out. Many will fall in battle, not because of random violence, but as a direct result of long-standing rebellion. This judgment is serious, but it is not the end of the story.

Immediately after this declaration, God reveals His plan for restoration. He promises to bring healing to the city—a promise that stands in sharp contrast to the destruction unfolding. This healing is not just physical; it includes spiritual renewal, emotional restoration, and national revival. God declares that He will forgive His people, cleanse them from sin, and lead them into a future filled with peace and truth. The message shifts from despair to hope, from punishment to promise.

The word translated as "health" in this passage is the Hebrew word *arukah*, which carries deep meaning. It comes from the root *arak*, meaning to arrange, prolong, or prepare. *Arukah* describes a healing that is complete, lasting, and intentional. It is not a quick fix or a temporary solution. Instead, it refers to a process of restoration that brings things back to their proper state. In the Bible, *arukah* is used to describe something that has been repaired and made whole again.

This promise of *arukah* is central to the hope God gives through Jeremiah. God assures His people that He will bring back those who were taken captive, rebuild the land, and restore Jerusalem as a place of divine favor. The city, once broken by sin and war, will become a symbol of God's mercy and power. Nations around the world will hear of its renewal and be amazed. The blessings poured out on Jerusalem will inspire reverence—not fear, but awe at God's goodness and grace.

This passage highlights three important spiritual truths:

- **Mercy After Judgment.** The order of events—judgment followed by healing—shows the rhythm of God's mercy. His anger is never random; it responds to persistent wrongdoing. But even in judgment, God's goal is redemption. As Jeremiah 29:11 says, "For I know the plans I have for you... plans for peace and not for evil, to give you a future and a hope." God's discipline is meant to correct and restore. His justice is always balanced by compassion.

- **Complete Restoration.** The healing God promises is full and complete. It includes physical safety, spiritual renewal, and the rebuilding of community. Jerusalem's restoration is not just about walls and buildings—it's about identity, purpose, and relationship with God. The people are not only freed from captivity; they are brought back into covenant with Him. Their sins are forgiven, their wounds are healed, and their future is secure. This kind of healing reflects the biblical view that body, soul, and society are all connected and restored together.

- **A Global Witness.** Jerusalem's renewal becomes a testimony to the world. As Ezekiel 36:23 says, **"I will vindicate the holiness of my great name... and the nations will know that I am the Lord."** The transformation of the city is not just for its people—it reveals God's character to everyone. His justice, mercy, and power are made visible through the restoration of His people. The city becomes a living example of what God can do, drawing others to worship and trust Him.

In conclusion, this passage from Jeremiah offers a powerful message of hope in the middle of despair. It shows that even when everything seems lost, God is still working—bringing justice, but also offering healing. The promise of *arukah* reminds us that God's restoration is deep, lasting, and complete. Jerusalem's story is not one of destruction, but of redemption. It is a testimony to the God who heals, forgives, and makes all things whole again.

Conclusion

As we come to the end of this study on *Healing in the Old Testament*, it becomes clear that healing in Scripture is much more than a physical event. Healing is connected to God's character, God's covenant, and God's desire to restore His people. The Old Testament shows that healing touches every part of life—body, mind, spirit, relationships, and community. It is never only about illness; it is about God bringing wholeness to what has been damaged or broken.

One of the strongest messages in the Old Testament is that God is the true source of healing. Sometimes God heals directly, through His power alone. Other times He heals through prophets, priests, prayers, or instructions. He may use natural means, rituals, or simple acts of obedience. But the point remains the same: healing comes from the God who created life. He is not far away from His people. He hears, sees, and responds to suffering. Whether healing happens quickly or slowly, whether it comes in dramatic ways or quiet ones, it always reflects God's love and care.

Healing is also closely connected to the covenant relationship. The covenant is not just a legal agreement; it is a bond of love and loyalty between

God and His people. God promises to bless and protect Israel, and the people promise to follow His ways. In many Old Testament passages, healing, protection, and long life are linked to obedience and trust. Sickness and hardship are sometimes linked to disobedience or injustice. However, the Old Testament also makes clear that not all suffering is punishment. Job's story especially reminds us that pain can come for reasons we do not understand. Still, the covenant gives God's people a foundation for hope, because God remains faithful even in their struggles.

A major theme throughout the Old Testament is that healing is holistic. Human beings are treated as whole persons. If the body suffers, the spirit suffers. If someone is excluded from the community because of illness, the emotional and social pain can be as great as the physical pain. This is why healing often includes more than physical recovery. It includes restoring someone to worship, to family, and to community life. It includes restoring dignity, hope, and identity. Healing is about bringing a person back into the fullness of life that God intends for them.

The Old Testament also shows that healing is not only individual; sometimes it is corporate. Entire families, tribes, and nations experience healing. God heals the land when the people turn away from sin. God restores the nation when they repent from idolatry and return to justice. Healing is tied to righteousness, mercy, and faithfulness. Where injustice and idolatry take root, suffering grows.

Where compassion and obedience take root, healing grows. This reminds us that healing is also a social responsibility. Communities are called to protect the weak, care for the sick, and act with fairness so that healing and peace can spread.

Stories of healing in the Old Testament show the personal side of suffering. Real men and women cry out to God. Some wait for years for relief. Some are healed suddenly, while others find comfort in God's presence rather than in physical recovery. These stories teach that healing is often a journey. It may involve prayer, patience, repentance, or faithful endurance. It may also involve mystery, because God does not always act in the way people expect. But in every story, God is near, even when His plans are not clear.

The prophets add another layer to the Old Testament's view of healing. They call the people to turn from sin, protect the poor, and return to God. They also speak of spiritual healing, where hearts are softened and lives are transformed. The prophets offer hope even in dark times. They promise that God will one day act in a powerful way to restore His people fully. This connects individual healings to a larger plan. God is not only concerned with one moment of suffering; He is guiding history toward a future of complete restoration.

The Book of Psalms gives us a close look at the emotional and spiritual nature of healing. The psalmists express fear, sadness, frustration, and confusion. Yet they also express trust, confidence, and praise. They teach us that prayer is part of healing. Even before anything changes on the outside, healing begins when a person turns to God honestly. The Psalms show that God welcomes our emotions and walks with us through them.

The laws about purity, community life, and care for the vulnerable also show that healing is a community process. People are expected to protect one another from harm, support those who are suffering, and make sure no one is left out. Priests examine those who are sick, rituals help people re-enter the community, and shared responsibility helps restore order and peace. Healing is not done in isolation. It involves family, leaders, neighbors, and the entire community of faith.

At the center of all this stands one truth: God desires to restore life. Healing is part of who God is. His compassion is deep and steady. His mercy is patient and strong. Whether through miracles, medicine, wise choices, or supportive relationships, healing is a sign of God's presence. The Old Testament does not promise a life without suffering, but it does promise that God is near to those who hurt and that He works continually to bring renewal.

Of course, the Old Testament is also honest about the mystery of suffering. Not every prayer is answered in the way a person hopes. Some questions remain unresolved. Books like Job and Ecclesiastes remind us that human understanding is limited. They teach us humility and trust. But even in these books, God remains active, just, and compassionate. Suffering never means abandonment.

The Old Testament ends with a message of hope. Healing is shown to be part of God's plan for His people over the long term. From the beginning, God did not intend for humans to live with sickness. The first time the word "healed" appears in the Bible is in Genesis 20:17, where God heals infertility. This connects back to Sarai in Genesis 11:30, where infertility is mentioned as the first physical illness recorded in human history.

This means that from the Garden of Eden, through the Flood, the Tower of Babel, and up to the time of Abram, the Bible does not mention any sickness among people. This detail gives strength to the words of the prophets, who spoke of a future when God would bring complete restoration and end the suffering that has affected humanity since this time.

This promise of healing still shapes how we think today. It teaches us to wait patiently in faith, to show compassion to others, and to trust that God's work of restoration is not yet finished.

In closing, healing in the Old Testament is a rich and powerful theme. It teaches that God heals the body, the heart, the spirit, the community, and even the land. It shows that healing is connected to justice, mercy, holiness, and faith. It calls people to trust God, pray honestly, and support one another. And it points toward a future where God's healing will be complete.

The Old Testament invites us to see healing not only as a moment but as a relationship—an ongoing walk with a God who cares, restores, and brings life. Even in times of pain, God is present. His desire to heal remains strong, and His promise to restore continues to give hope. This is the heart of healing in the Old Testament: the faithful love of God meeting the broken places of life and bringing wholeness, peace, and renewal.

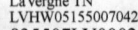

www.ingramcontent.com/pod-product-compliance
Lightning Source LLC
LaVergne TN
LVHW051550070426
835507LV00021B/2512